Plagues and the Paradox of Progress

Plagues and the Paradox of Progress

Why the World Is Getting Healthier in Worrisome Ways

Thomas J. Bollyky

A Council on Foreign Relations Book
The MIT Press
Cambridge, Massachusetts
London, England

This book was set in Stone Serif by Westchester Publishing Services. Printed and bound in the United States of America.

Library of Congress Cataloging-in-Publication Data

Names: Bollyky, Thomas J., author.
Title: Plagues and the paradox of progress : why the world is getting healthier in worrisome ways / Thomas J. Bollyky.
Description: Cambridge, MA : The MIT Press, [2018] | Includes bibliographical references and index.
Identifiers: LCCN 2017059434 | ISBN 9780262038454 (hardcover : alk. paper)
Subjects: | MESH: Global Health—trends | Communicable Diseases—history | Disease Eradication | Noncommunicable Diseases | Health Status Disparities—trends | Socioeconomic Factors
Classification: LCC RA418 | NLM WA 530.1 | DDC 362.1—dc23 LC record available at https://lccn.loc.gov/2017059434

10 9 8 7 6 5 4 3 2 1

To my daughters and son, for whom the world should simply get better. And to my wife and their mother, who makes that seem possible.

Contents

Preface

There was a little figure plump,
For every little knoll ...
Playmates, and holidays, and nuts,
And visions vast and small
Strange that the feet so precious charged
Should reach so small a goal!"
—Emily Dickinson, "Time and Eternity"

In New England, where I grew up, the history of four hundred years of disease and development is written in stone. The landscape is crossed with dry stonewalls, testimony to backbreaking hours spent transforming forests and wilderness into fields and pastures. Old mills, dams, canal locks, and factories—the foundations of industrialization—still dot the landscape. But it is the headstones in churchyards and old family plots that provide perhaps the most direct, human connection to that past.

One such old family cemetery plot was just down the street, near my school bus stop. For years, I occasionally stopped to look at the names and dates engraved on the headstones. The children outnumbered the adults buried in this small plot and I recall several stones for infants who never made it past their first month. By the time I completed elementary school, I was older than most of the occupants of that cemetery plot. Yet, I did not experience the death of a friend or playmate until college. Not only did I survive childhood, but nearly all of my peers did too.

My good fortune is a relatively recent development. In 1880, the date listed on the most recent grave in that plot, twenty-two out of every one hundred infants in the United States died before their first birthday and

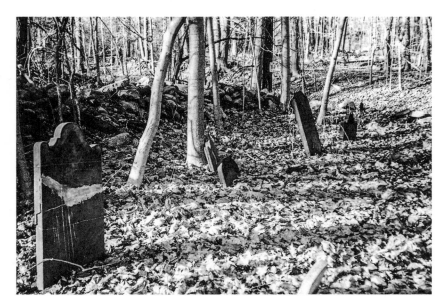

Figure 0.1
Farms Road Cemetery. Photo: Richard Roberts, 2004. Courtesy of the Stamford
Historical Society.

many more were stricken with serious illness. The survival rates for African-
American children were worse.[1] The United States was not poor in 1880, not
even by today's standards.[2] The country was industrializing, particularly in
New England, and the nation experienced strong economic growth in the
two decades before the US Civil War. Americans were literate and well fed
relative to the citizens of other nations. And yet, US life expectancy at birth
had only gotten worse.[3]

The dominant killers of infants and children in the United States in
1880 were bacteria, viruses, parasites, and protozoa that led to infectious
diseases, and human responses to those diseases. Terrifying epidemics of
smallpox, yellow fever, and typhoid motivated the governments of the
United States and modernizing nations in Europe to promote measures
like smallpox vaccination and quarantine. But the everyday infectious diseases like pneumonia, measles, dysentery, scarlet fever, and tuberculosis kept
coming, waging their unrelenting assault on American children. Effective
medicines for those diseases would not be invented for decades. A visit

from a doctor or a remedy bought from pharmacy was as likely to harm a child as help.[4]

The accounts of children's illnesses and their treatment constitute a significant part of nineteenth-century American women's writings about motherhood. Each new developmental stage, from feeding to teething to weaning, seemed to bring new risks of infection. Parents could do little but live in constant fear that their children would die, so they had more babies in the hopes that some might live.[5] The good health that my siblings, the other neighborhood children, and I enjoyed a hundred years later, living in that same community, must have seemed unthinkable.

By the time I reached college, my concerns with disease and its effects on societies were with the present, not the past. An internship at the New York City Department of Health at the height of the city's HIV/AIDS crisis demonstrated in real time the consequences of epidemics and human responses to them. That searing experience moved me to forgo lab science after finishing my degree and to devote my career to global health, law, and policy.

I first learned about the great histories of parasites, viruses, and other infectious diseases when my brother Paul returned home from college and announced a career change of his own: he no longer wanted to be an architect. He had just finished William McNeill's *Plagues and Peoples*, which tells the story of how encounters with infectious diseases have shaped the course of human history, enabling some conquests while dooming others, changing the fortunes of empires, and determining the religious beliefs and cultures of peoples. The book offered a new way of viewing the world, and it resonated with my brother. That interest evolved into a vocation; my brother became an infectious disease doctor. For his fortieth birthday, I cold-called Professor McNeill, who was then 94 years old and semiretired in Connecticut, and asked if he would sign and dedicate a copy of his book. He kindly agreed, and that first edition sits on my brother's shelf, inscribed in shaky script: "a book you know well."

It is easy to be taken with McNeill's landmark book and the other great histories of infectious disease. They tell fascinating stories about the role of microbes in the Spanish conquest of Latin America, the collapse of feudalism, the invention of the printing press, and the delayed colonization of Africa. These books make for excellent dinner party conversation (at my house at least). It is hard to resist Hans Zinsser's description, in his 1935 book, *Rats, Lice, and History*, of infectious disease research as swashbuckling affairs in exotic lands:

> Infectious disease is one of the few genuine adventures left in the world. The dragons are all dead and the lance grows rusty in the chimney corner. ... About the only sporting proposition that remains unimpaired by the relentless domestication of a once free-living human species is the war against those ferocious little fellow creatures, which lurk in the dark corners and stalk us in the bodies of rats, mice and all kinds of domestic animals; which fly and crawl with the insects, and waylay us in our food and drink and even in our love.[6]

It was only in writing this book about the ways in which changes in global health are shaping the modern world that I came to think again about the role of infectious diseases in the past. McNeill argued that the impact of infectious diseases on the course of world events goes beyond good tales about the thwarted ambitions of kings and captains, which still holds true today. Understanding the role of plagues and parasites in world affairs still provides key insights into the evolution of the state, the growth and geography of cities, the disparate fortunes of national economies, and the reasons why people migrate. This book tells that story, but it is not about the rise or resurgence of plagues, pestilence, and parasites. It is the story of their decline. This book explores the manner and consequences of that decline, first in New England and the other wealthy, industrialized regions of North America and Europe and eventually in many of the world's poorest nations. In other words, this book picks up where *Plagues and Peoples* left off.

Miracles have occurred in the global fight against infectious disease, especially in the last fifteen years. Deaths from malaria and tuberculosis have roughly halved. In 2003, 100,000 people in sub-Saharan Africa with HIV/AIDS were on lifesaving treatment; today, more than 10 million people are. The great killers of children—pneumonia, diarrheal diseases, measles, whooping cough, and diphtheria—are receding. The once fearsome scourges of polio and Guinea worm are on the verge of extinction, where they will join smallpox on the short list of diseases that humankind has successfully eradicated. To be sure, far too many children and adults still die each year from HIV/AIDS, tuberculosis, malaria, and other infectious diseases. The decline in plagues and parasites has not been uninterrupted, and it is not guaranteed to continue. Recent outbreaks of the Ebola and Zika viruses are reminders that the risk of pandemics remains ever present and worthy of our constant vigilance. But just because the war on microbes is far from over should not obscure the fact that we are in the midst of a dramatic change in the lived human experience.

For the first time in recorded history, parasites, viruses, bacteria, and other infectious diseases are not the leading cause of death and disability in any region of the world. Eleven thousand fewer children under the age of five die each day from infectious diseases than did twenty-five years ago. The infant mortality rate in the Central African Republic is the highest in the world, but it is half of what it was in 1960 and roughly a third of what it was in the United States in 1880. People are living longer and fewer mothers are giving birth to many children in the hopes that some might survive.

In the past, declines in infectious diseases and longer, healthier lives were a path to prosperity and inclusion. The economist Robert Gordon has argued that "the historic decline in infant mortality centered in the six-decade period of 1890–1950 is one of the most important single facts in the history of American economic growth."[7] US cities, which had staggered against repeated waves of infection, began to flourish. With the improvement in child survival and declining fertility, the rate of women's participation in the workforce more than doubled, from 12 percent in 1870 to 26 percent in 1940. Girls' literacy rates improved, and they attended school in greater numbers, with fewer obligations to assist their mothers in caring for their many siblings. Child mortality and school attendance for African Americans continued to lag behind whites, but also improved dramatically.

The early results of the more recent global declines in infectious diseases and child mortality have not been as good. Longer lives in many countries have not been accompanied by the same economic growth, job opportunities, and better governance that occurred with those changes in today's wealthy nations. These muted gains are not simply the consequence of hopeless poverty and political instability in the countries where the recent declines in infectious diseases have occurred. China was among the world's poorest countries and on the cusp of famine and cultural revolution when that country began a dramatic campaign against infectious diseases that set the stage for it to emerge as one of the great global economic powers.

The different outcomes of progress against infectious disease are due, instead, to the different ways progress has occurred and the global moment at which it is now happening. Nearly two-thirds of the gains in life expectancy that have occurred in the United States since 1880 predated the availability of most treatments for infectious diseases.[8] Medical innovations and

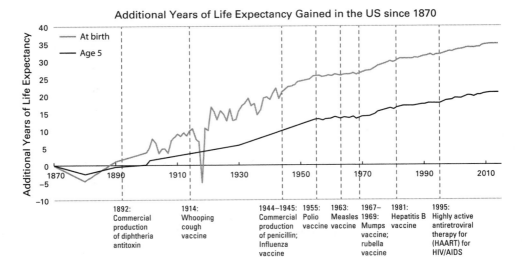

Figure 0.2
Data sources: US Census Bureau, CDC, Proquest.

foreign aid are playing a greater role now, which has enabled these more recent reductions in plagues and parasites to occur without the gradual social, political, and public health reforms needed to overcome infectious diseases in the past. This approach has prevented millions of unnecessary deaths, but it has not been a panacea for poorer nations and there have been some unintended consequences. One such consequence is that many poorer nations are experiencing increases in noncommunicable diseases like cancers, heart disease, and diabetes that are three to four times faster than have ever been seen in most wealthy nations. Another consequence is the advent of a new phenomenon in human history: poor world cities. Urban areas in lower-income nations are rapidly growing beyond the bounds of their infrastructure, even without the promise of factory jobs to lure farm hands away from their fields and toward the city lights.

These unintended consequences are exacerbated by factors that most rich countries did not encounter when reducing their burden of plagues, parasites, and viruses. Climate change and increased hostility to trade and immigration in wealthy nations has left poorer countries less equipped to take advantage of the opportunities that accompany declining rates of infectious diseases, and ill-positioned to cope with the resulting challenges. At the same time, many national governments, philanthropies, and international institutions have been slow to adjust to a world in which infectious disease is no longer the dominant problem it once was. The consequences of these challenges and the failure to address them adequately are worrisome and are reverberating across the world's economic, political, and security landscape.

In short, our recent progress against infectious diseases is a paradox. The historic health achievements of the past decades are remaking a world that is both worrisome and full of unprecedented opportunities. Whether the peril or promise of progress prevails depends on what we do next. Explaining why this is happening and the challenges that lie ahead is the task of this book.

This paradox in the recent progress against infectious diseases has deep roots and far-reaching implications. As a result, this book is necessarily multidisciplinary, a mix of science, history, and international affairs intended for a broad audience. It draws on my own work, often with coauthors, but also on the ideas and scholarship of many others. That list starts with William McNeill, Hans Zinsser, Paul de Kruif, and other authors of the classic histories of infectious diseases, and also includes subsequent scholars who have benefited from microbiological advances that are improving much of what we know about infectious diseases past and present. The price of genetic sequencing has fallen significantly in recent years and there have been dramatic improvements in the ability of researchers to extract and sequence DNA from once-unpromising sources like medieval teeth, ancient bone fragments, Hungarian mummy tissue, and fossilized gorilla feces.[9] These developments have greatly increased researchers' ability to trace the origin, evolution, and impact of microbes in human history.[10]

In exploring the role that the decline of infectious diseases plays in urbanization, the evolution of the modern state, economic development, migration, and other areas, this book pulls from diverse sources, including the work of many economists and epidemiologists, historians and health workers. Those on whose research I have relied are cited in the text where possible, and without exception in the endnotes. In some sections, I make my case in numbers, depicted in graphs. In each of those instances, I explain the source of those data and how they contribute to the argument of the book: that the ongoing decline in infectious diseases is as consequential as their rise. And, like those great histories of infectious diseases, this book has some good stories to tell, too.

We are in an era of great and welcome progress in the global fight against infectious disease. That fight must continue and we should continue to invest in it. But we must also recognize that making this progress against plagues and parasites has brought about new and unintended challenges, as important progress often does. For us to seize the opportunities and prosperity that came with health improvements in the past, these emerging challenges must be recognized and overcome. Failing to do so may undermine or reverse hard-fought improvements in health and living standards that have been achieved in recent decades.

This book is not just about the role of plagues in the sweep of history, but the countless lives that were lost, one by one, to those diseases, and the precious opportunities to be gained when those lives are saved in an environment where individuals can take advantage of those opportunities. The aim of this book is to accomplish what William McNeill's classic book *Plagues and Peoples* has done: to move its readers to see what is happening in the world differently and to be motivated to do something about it.

Introduction

Infectious disease which antedated the emergence of humankind will last as long as humanity itself, and will surely remain, as it has been hitherto, one of the fundamental parameters and determinants of human history.
—William H. McNeill, *Plagues and Peoples*

No other development over the last hundred years—not world wars, not the internet, not the spread of democracy—has had as widespread and transformative an impact on the human experience as the decline in infectious diseases. This book is about the paradox of that progress in the long fight against parasites, viruses, and other plagues: the world is getting better in ways that should make us worry.

The slow decline in the death and disability from infectious diseases began 250 years ago with the Enlightenment and the Industrial Revolution in Northern Europe and spread to the United States and other countries with deep European roots. After World War II, this trend began to accelerate and extend globally and, in recent years, has reached even the poorest countries. The consequences of this expanded control of infectious disease are hard to overstate.

As recently as sixty years ago, most developing nations were still subject to the cycle of low life expectancy and high birth rates that have characterized humankind for millennia.[1] In 1950, one out of five children still perished before their fifth birthday in nearly one hundred countries, including almost every nation in sub-Saharan Africa, South Asia, and Southeast Asia. The average life expectancy of a baby born in these nations was 42 years. With so many dying young, few children received a formal education, and most grew up to live lives similar to those of their parents and the generations before them: in rural settings and engaged in subsistence farming. There was a thirty-three-year difference between the average life expectancy in Northern Europe (70 years old) and sub-Saharan Africa (37 years old).

Lower-income nations have significantly narrowed these gaps since the 1950s. By 2015, the average baby born in a developing country was expected to live to 70. The number of countries where one out of five children perish under the age of five is now zero. With fewer children and adolescents dying, investment in education in many lower-income nations has dramatically improved. The average adult in Bangladesh, Haiti, and Zambia now has more years of schooling than the average adult in France or Italy did in 1960.[2] Agriculture no longer employs the majority of people in most regions of the world. Just over half of those living in developing countries now reside in a city. The total number of people in lower-income nations has expanded from 1.7 billion in 1950 to 6.1 billion in 2015. Despite this population increase, per-capita incomes in developing nations have grown and extreme poverty has declined, driven by increased global trade, Asian manufacturing, and rising commodity prices. By 2015, the gap in life expectancy between Northern Europe and sub-Saharan Africa had shrunk by ten years.

All this progress that has been achieved against plagues and parasites is one of the great achievements of humankind, but it is also spurring new and daunting challenges. When richer countries took on the scourge of infectious diseases, few advanced medicines were available. Their tools, therefore, included social controls, like quarantines, and investments in effective water and sewage systems. These tools required or led to more responsive governments and capable health-care systems, which in turn helped advance the prosperity of those nations.

In contrast, the recent gains in infectious disease control in many lower-income nations have been more dependent on international aid and effective medical technologies.[3] As a result, the decline in infectious disease in many (but by no means all) lower-income nations has not been accompanied by the same improvements in personal wealth, health care, responsive governments, and employment opportunities that accompanied those changes in today's wealthier nations. In the absence of those broader improvements, many emerging economies are struggling to cope with the demographic changes that have occurred with the decline of infectious diseases—unprecedented urbanization and a rapid rise in the number of working-age adults. At the same time, the world is changing, with wealthy nations adopting trade and immigration policies that are much less accommodating of these demographic changes happening in poorer nations. Climate change is making it harder for farmers and pastoralists in many regions to earn a living, adding to the pressure for them to migrate. If donors and international institutions remain slow to respond to these emerging challenges, there could be dire consequences that resound through the world's economic, political, and security landscape.

To explain the cause for concern, this book must convince you of three insights: first, that infectious diseases are indeed declining; second, that the threat of infectious diseases and the efforts to overcome that threat have played and will continue to play an important role in shaping the modern world; and third, that the way infectious diseases are declining in recent decades is different from how they have declined in the past, and that difference, when combined with broader global changes, is producing deeply worrisome consequences for the future. I outline these arguments briefly in this introduction, but we will explore them in depth in the pages that follow.

The Age-Old Balance between Host and Parasite

The notion that infectious diseases are in decline may be hard to believe. There are still 36.7 million people worldwide living with HIV/AIDS. More than six million people were newly infected with tuberculosis in 2016. The World Health Organization estimates that roughly 185,000 people die annually from neglected tropical diseases.[4] Outbreaks of exotic parasites, bacterial blights, and obscure tropical viruses dominate the news. Deservedly, much attention has been given to the lives lost and children disabled in high-profile epidemics of influenza, severe acute respiratory syndrome (SARS), and the Ebola and Zika viruses. Reports of smaller outbreaks of well-known infections and encounters with new diseases continue to occur regularly.[5] People and plagues, McNeill wrote, exist in "an age-old balance between host and parasite"; and those infectious diseases will remain "a permanent feature of human (and all multi-cellular forms of) life."[6]

New and previously unknown infectious diseases are likely to remain an ever-present threat to human life. Viruses, such as Ebola or avian influenza, continue to jump from animals to humans, evolve, and intermingle in ways that make them deadlier and more prone to spread. Overuse of existing drugs and underinvestment in new ones are producing drug-resistant strains of fungi, protozoa, tuberculosis, and other bacteria, making routine medical care more dangerous. These emerging and treatment-resistant pathogens easily cross national boundaries, given increases in global trade, faster travel, and rising global temperatures (resulting in warmer, more virus-friendly climates).[7] The risk of another great pandemic of infectious disease—similar to the Black Death of bubonic plague in the fourteenth century, cholera in the nineteenth century, influenza in 1918–19, or HIV/AIDS—is not behind us.

Given our increasingly intertwined world, these threats are still worthy of serious concern, even if they are not entirely new. Infectious disease has accompanied trade since at least 430 BCE, when a plague brought by infected rats aboard a trading ship killed a third of the population of Athens. Cholera spread in the nineteenth century via railways across North America and on steamships to the United Kingdom and the rest of Europe.[8] Resistant strains of bacteria predated the discovery of the first antibiotics.[9] Climate change allowed malaria to expand out of Africa centuries ago and likely influenced all three major pandemics of bubonic plague, including the Black Death of the Middle Ages.[10] New risks such as synthetic, man-made viruses may yet emerge, but for now, the differences between the contribution of globalization, climate change, and drug resistance to today's infectious disease threats and those of the past are largely matters of degree, not kind. The long-standing process of managing these threats remains deeply important.

But that ongoing threat should not blind us to what has changed. In the last few decades—for the first time in recorded human history—infectious diseases have declined significantly, even in the poorest populations. According to the University of Washington's Institute for Health Metrics and Evaluation, a leading source of data on global health, infectious diseases now account for less than 8 percent of the death and disability in most regions of the world, including many lower-income and tropical regions such as the Middle East and North Africa, and Latin America and the Caribbean. There are only two exceptions. The first is South Asia, which includes India, Pakistan, and more impoverished nations like Bangladesh and Nepal; infectious diseases are responsible for roughly one-fifth of the health burden in that region. The second is sub-Saharan Africa, where plagues and parasites stopped being the cause of the majority of death and disability in 2011. Four years later, that rate fell to less than 44 percent in this poorest of geographic regions.

The long-term declines in infectious diseases have proven durable, even amid outbreaks and epidemics of new and reemerging infections. HIV/AIDS has exacted a terrible toll, disproportionately in sub-Saharan Africa. At its peak in 2005, the disease killed 1.8 million people annually. With the efforts of the US government and other donors and partners to expand access to antiretroviral treatment and prevent HIV/AIDS transmission from mothers to their infants, death rates from the disease dropped 42 percent in a decade. Even in countries with the highest rates of HIV/AIDS infection, such as Botswana, average life expectancy rates have bounced back and now exceed pre-epidemic levels.

The recent progress and resilience against HIV/AIDS and other infectious diseases reflect the tireless, coordinated efforts of many. The relative success of their efforts was not a foregone conclusion, and there is much more left to do, especially in the poorest countries. Population growth, urbanization, and the decline of endemic infectious diseases in many countries have increased the risks of future outbreaks and epidemics by bringing larger numbers of people without prior exposure to infections into closer contact with each other. The risks of emerging infections, antibiotic resistance, and bioterrorism remain important, and preparing for future pandemics requires sustained global investment.

But the continued threat of microbes to humankind should not obscure the overall decline in rates of infectious disease any more than a terrible snowstorm would disprove the otherwise steady rise in global temperatures. Indeed, as with climate change and extreme weather events, there may be ties between the falling global rates of everyday plagues and parasites and the heightened risk of occasional infectious disease outbreaks. The decline in infectious diseases is unprecedented and sustained, and it is transforming lower-income countries. Most of that transformation has happened in just the last few decades. The effects extend beyond longer lives and less suffering, to the growth and the geography of cities and to shifts in global economic power and patterns of human migration. Not all these changes have been positive.

Determinants of History, Agents of Human Tragedy

To understand how and why the decline of infectious diseases is reshaping the world, for good and for ill, we need to return to McNeill. He argued in *Plagues and Peoples* that infectious diseases have been "one of the fundamental parameters and determinants of human history." Subsequent scholars have joined McNeill in the observation that the power of microbes has often extended beyond their death toll.[11] Three traits account for the outsized influence of infectious diseases over human history.

First, infectious diseases, by definition, can spread. That transmission can occur from person to person or indirectly through an insect or animal intermediary such as a mosquito or rat. The risk of transmission is greatest in settlements and with activities that bring large numbers of people into close contact. For this reason, encounters with infectious disease have played a key role in the evolution of cities, the expansion of trading routes, the conduct of war, and participation in pilgrimages. Again, it is hard to improve on Zinsser:

> Swords and lances, arrows, machine guns, and even high explosives have had less power over the fates of the nations than the typhus louse, the plague flea, and the yellow fever mosquito. Civilizations have retreated from the plasmodium of malaria, and armies have crumbled into rabbles under the onslaught of cholera spirilla, or of dysentery and typhoid bacilli. Huge areas have been devastated by the trypanosome that travels on the wings of the tsetse fly, and generations have been harassed by the syphilis of a courtier. War and conquest and that herd existence which is an accompaniment of what we call civilization have merely set the stage for these most powerful agents of human tragedy.[12]

Second, infectious diseases disproportionately affect previously unexposed people. When plagues and parasites do not kill, survivors are often left with life-long immunity to a reoccurrence of the disease. Many histories of infectious disease have focused on ways in which populations without that prior immunity have borne the brunt of the microbes that accompanied invading armies, trade caravans, and explorers. The risk that plagues and parasites pose for people without prior immunity is also why many infectious diseases disproportionately affect children. Infectious diseases have kept rates of child mortality high throughout most of human history, which has both led mothers to have more children in order to compensate for those who might be lost and undercut the incentive for families to invest in their young. Those consequences, in turn, have had profound implications for the role of women in societies, education rates, and the composition of labor forces.

The third reason for the outsized role of infectious disease in human history is that their prevention and control depends on the cooperation of people and governments. Individuals, households, communities, and nations cannot isolate themselves from the risk of infectious disease for long, and can do so only at great cost.[13] Measures to prevent and control infectious disease can succeed and be sustained only if our neighbors, other communities, and national governments undertake those measures too. The Nobel Laureate Joshua Lederberg once aptly wrote: "The microbe that felled one child in a distant continent yesterday can reach yours today and seed a global pandemic tomorrow."[14]

Other threats to human health, such as tobacco products, illicit drugs, and air pollution, can also cross national borders and require a collective response to be effective. But infectious diseases predate these other concerns as the first global problem that nation-states realized could not be solved without international cooperation. The words that the English political theorist Leonard S. Woolf wrote in 1916 still ring true: "The conflict fought by the theory of national independence, isolation, and national interests against the facts of international life and international interests has nowhere shown itself more persistently and clearly than in the struggle of human beings against the scourges of cholera, plague, and other epidemic diseases."[15] Infectious diseases have been a particularly good motivator of collective action because of the disproportionate threat they pose to populations without prior exposure, the dread that these diseases inspire, and the economic losses that may result when epidemics disrupt international trade and travel.[16]

The Different Paths to Progress

Infectious diseases forced governments to assume greater administrative power and authority over the practices of their citizens and commercial enterprises. The understanding that some diseases were contagious dates back to the Bible, which includes detailed rules for isolating lepers in their homes.[17] With the first major Black Death epidemic in the fourteenth century, local authorities in Venice and Florence applied that Old Testament practice of forced isolation to persons in transit.[18] The word *quarantine* derives from *quaranta giorni*, which means "forty days" in Italian. Renaissance-era governments adopted other public health innovations to cope with epidemics as well: requiring civil registration of citizens and forming the first municipal boards of health. These measures represented a significant expansion of state authority and were copied by other countries struggling to cope with outbreaks of plague and parasites.[19]

When the threat of epidemics involved cholera and other microbial threats where quarantine was ineffective, governments adapted, expanding again on examples from the past. Jewish, Hindu, and Islamic laws include rules on bodily cleanliness and the handling of food and water. The Romans built an elaborate network of aqueducts, underground channels, and pipes to drain the surrounding swamps, which stemmed the tide of malaria and provided sanitation and drinking water.[20] Under pressure from social reformers and angry citizen mobs, governments of wealthy countries in the nineteenth century constructed water and waste-management systems, adopted housing codes and food regulations, promoted personal hygiene, and entered into the first international health treaties to contain epidemic threats.[21]

Most of the gains in infectious disease control in higher-income nations occurred before the invention of effective medical treatments for those diseases. The precise mix of measures undertaken varied by disease and by country, as did the rate of the progress.[22] The path to progress against pestilence was not linear; countries suffered reversals and important innovations, such as the germ theory of disease, took decades to be widely adopted.[23] But many of the nations that experienced significant, long-term declines in plagues and parasites shared common themes: increased industrialization and a rising middle class, the advent of trade unions and better women's education, and the establishment of public health laws and more responsive government institutions.[24] In some cases, control of infectious disease was largely the result of changes such as rising incomes and increased access to education. In others, infectious disease control spurred investment in sanitation, housing laws, and municipal infrastructure that then had broader societal and economic benefits for now-wealthy nations. In these ways, the slow process of infectious disease control both required and allowed many governments to improve their functioning. That commitment cannot flag; where developed countries have failed to sustain their investments in controlling plagues and parasites, they have suffered resurgences of diseases such as tuberculosis.[25]

The recent decline in plagues, viruses, and parasites in poorer countries is just as important as those past health improvements were in now-wealthy nations. But the efforts to control infectious disease threats in many lower-income nations are not driving the same social reform and investment in municipal, national, and international governance as those efforts did decades ago. The heavy burden of plagues, viruses, and parasites is being overcome in the cities of many lower-income nations without effective housing laws, adequate municipal water and sewage systems, and the economic infrastructure needed to attract factories that can put migrants to work. The particular risk that infectious diseases pose to previously unexposed peoples, particularly infants and children, is being surmounted without commensurate improvements in public health and in the status of women.

Why Worry in the Age of Miracles?

Michael Elliott, the late journalist and former CEO of the ONE Campaign, rightly called this era in global health "the age of miracles."[26] Better infectious disease control in lower-income nations has saved millions of children and infants who otherwise would have perished or lived a life of infirmity.

In too many countries, however, too little is being done to ensure that the children and infants surviving to adulthood find employment opportunities and adequate health systems to accommodate their needs as adults. The World Bank estimates that the working-age population (more than 15 years old) in developing countries will increase by 2.1 billion by 2050. Unless current national employment rates improve, that will mean nearly 900 million more young adults without work.[27] Rates of chronic diseases that are most associated with affluent nations, such as heart disease, cancer, and diabetes, are rising fast in lower-income countries without capable health-care systems to prevent and manage these diseases. The growth of cities in many poorer nations is historically unprecedented, far outpacing their urban economies and infrastructure. For the first time in history, the existence of large cities is not necessarily indicative of prosperity and good governance. Congested metropolises and the lack of formal employment for rising youth populations threaten to breed instability. Climate change and increased hostility to trade and immigration in wealthy nations are exacerbating the situation by leaving poorer nations with fewer avenues for expanding job opportunities and restricting the ability of their citizens to move elsewhere. It is not hard to envision a scenario where the next several decades are less peaceful than the last.

A Worrisome Future Is Not Inevitable

The story of the decline in infectious diseases threatens to be as consequential as the history of their rise. It deserves to be recognized and treated as such. But a dire future is not inevitable. This book is not a treatise on overpopulation in developing countries or how the world would have been better off forgoing investment in global health. The planet does not thrive when the sickest are permitted to die off, but rather when they are able to improve their lives. Efforts to reduce infectious disease, early death, and unnecessary suffering in lower-income countries should continue. National governments, donors, and intergovernmental institutions should do everything possible to accelerate that process.

More people need not mean more people who are poor. Reductions in infectious disease can accelerate economic growth and better governance when accompanied by improvements in educational quality, infrastructure, and formal employment opportunities. Countries as diverse as Brazil, Iran, and Saudi Arabia have achieved fertility declines without resorting to draconian forms of population control. Despite long-standing fears and predictions to the contrary, innovations in agricultural production in the twentieth century have continued to enable it to exceed the rate of population growth.

But rejection of neo-Malthusian fears about hordes of people breeding in poorer nations does not mean we should ignore the new challenges emerging as a result of the progress made in the fight against infectious diseases. We should not assume that poor countries can or will follow the same path as wealthier nations.

Once, it was the more advanced nations of the world that were more disease-ridden. The disproportionate number of deaths from plagues and parasites in impoverished tropical and subtropical nations is a recent development in human history. Chapter 1 tells the story of how that changed, the link between the history of infectious diseases and agriculture, trade, urbanization, and humankind's other civilizing habits, and the long, slow route that wealthy nations took to better health. This chapter opens in South Africa in 2003, amid a raging HIV/AIDS epidemic. It is the moment when the gap between the incidence of infectious disease in the poorest nations and the wealthiest ones was arguably the largest in recorded human history.

The next four chapters describe the way that plagues and parasites have declined more recently in poorer nations, the different paths that this progress has taken, and the consequences. Each chapter focuses on a theme and uses case studies of particular diseases and countries to explore that theme.

Chapter 2 starts with diseases of conquest and colony: smallpox and malaria. The theme of this chapter is the link between infectious disease, foreign aid, and the state. It examines the military and colonial origins of the global disease eradication campaigns in the 1950s and their influence on the disease-specific, technology-driven strategies used to reduce the plagues and parasites in poorer nations. This approach has proved remarkably successful in addressing the targeted infectious diseases, but has not been accompanied by the broad improvements in responsive and more capable governments that occurred with the control of everyday infectious diseases in many wealthy nations. When combined with rapid population growth, urbanization, and more adults, the underdeveloped health-care systems in poor countries are straining to cope with the threat of new and emerging infections like Ebola and an unprecedented increase in noncommunicable diseases.

Chapter 3 turns to the diseases of childhood—measles and other respiratory diseases—that disproportionately affect children once they become endemic. The theme of this chapter is the link between infectious disease and economies. It starts with an audacious campaign launched in 1982 to extend childhood immunizations to the poorest regions of the world in just eight years. It then considers how the decline in mortality from childhood diseases helped transform the economic fortunes of some formerly poor countries in the space of just a few decades. This chapter also explains why the economic opportunity afforded by that decline in infectious disease is fleeting and potentially perilous. That story features China and Kenya.

Chapter 4 considers the diseases of settlement—tuberculosis, and cholera and other intestinal diseases—that rose to prominence in the first industrializing cities of Europe and America. The theme of this chapter is the link between infectious disease and urbanization. Frugal innovations to tackle these diseases have helped shift the geography and growth of mega-cities, a phenomenon once reserved for wealthy nations, but now found most often in lower-income countries. This chapter begins on the busy streets of Dhaka, Bangladesh, the most densely populated city on earth.

Chapter 5 addresses the diseases of place—meningitis and other neglected infectious and parasitic diseases—that occur almost exclusively in the poorest and most ecologically challenged regions of the world. These diseases have been the targets of heroic international health campaigns in the last fifteen years and are starting to decline. The infants and children saved by these recent health improvements are now starting to reach adulthood and to do what many of the beneficiaries of infectious disease control have always done: emigrate. The theme of this chapter is infectious disease and migration, and it focuses on Niger and Ireland.

The sixth and concluding chapter of this book opens with the story of William H. Stewart and one of the most famous, widely used, and erroneously attributed quotes in modern medicine. This chapter explains how the statement Stewart actually made is a useful frame for thinking about policy recommendations to build a world that continues to get better, just in less worrisome ways.

There is a future for lower-income nations that includes more inclusive economic growth, smart investments in health-care systems and education, freer trade, continued advances in technology, sustainable agricultural production, and better governance. Only the governments of those countries and the people who live there can realize that potential future. But foreign aid agencies, philanthropists, and the private sector can do much more to help those countries sustainably tackle their crushing demographic challenges. This book lays out that agenda, but to adopt and implement those solutions effectively we need a greater understanding of the nature and basic history of the problem and where and why it is occurring. That is the task of the next several chapters of this book.

1 How the World Starts Getting Better

Where are the drugs? That's where they are, the drugs are where the disease is not. And where is the disease? The disease is where the drugs are not.
—Dr. Peter Mugyenyi, Durban AIDS Conference, 2000

"I have an idea."

It was my first day of work at the AIDS Law Project, a nongovernmental organization based in Johannesburg, South Africa. I was fresh out of law school, eager to contribute. So when my new boss asked at the weekly staff meeting if anyone knew how to safely get a syringe of the drug Nevirapine to a woman about to give birth in a rural part of the country, I volunteered.

The intended recipient of that syringe, S,[1] was an expecting first-time mother and one of the four million South Africans living with HIV/AIDS in 2001.[2] One out of every four women at a public antenatal clinic tested positive for the disease that year, and S was one of them.[3] A fetus does not generally contract HIV in the womb, but an estimated 70,000 infants in South Africa at that time caught the virus each year when exposed to their mother's blood in childbirth or during breastfeeding. In her eighth month of pregnancy, S learned that she had HIV and that her baby was also at risk. S heard on the television that there was a medicine that could stop her baby from getting the disease, but that it was not available in South Africa. S spent two weeks, heavily pregnant and squeezed into hot, crowded minibuses, traveling the dusty, bumpy roads between NGO clinics and faith-based institutions, begging for someone to tell her how she could save her unborn daughter. A tip from a nun led to a hotline, which led to a referral to us. My boss managed to get the correct dose of Nevirapine from a physician friend. Now we just needed to get it to S before she went into labor, which could happen at any moment.

S and her unborn daughter were victims of geography and bad luck. S had had sex with only a single partner, a young man from her township, but in 2001, South Africa was a country where roughly one out of five adults was HIV positive. In 1996, the development of a three-drug combination of antiretroviral medicines transformed HIV/AIDS from a terrible killer to a manageable chronic condition in rich nations. Thabo Mbeki, South Africa's then-president, recognized AIDS as a serious threat, but denied the over-whelming scientific consensus that HIV caused the disease. He insisted on finding a uniquely African solution to the epidemic rather than becom-ing dependent on the wares of Western drug companies.[4] With a deeply loyal health minister, Manto Tshabalala-Msimang, and no viable opposi-tion party to the ruling African National Congress, the rest of the govern-ment fell in line. The South African government refused to provide access to Nevirapine, even when its manufacturer donated it, and other patented HIV drugs were far too expensive for patients like S to buy out of pocket. In 2001, more South Africans were dying in middle age, mostly from HIV/AIDS, than in their sixties and seventies.[5]

At least effective medicines for HIV existed. The burden from other infectious diseases, such as malaria and tuberculosis, was also high in South Africa and the sub-Saharan Africa region. Treatments for many of these other infectious diseases, when they existed, dated back to colonial times or were repurposed veterinary medicines and often toxic.[6] In nations that the World Bank defined as high-income in 2001, only 6 percent of the deaths were due to infectious diseases. But in sub-Saharan Africa, fifty-four out of every hundred deaths were still caused by the same infectious diseases that, with the exception of HIV/AIDS (a relatively new disease), had plagued humankind for millennia.[7]

After that staff meeting, I went to the kitchen area. I broke off a piece of the packing foam that came with the organization's new toaster and brought it to my new office. The syringe included a plastic sleeve to protect the needle, but it needed to be held firm without depressing the plunger. I dug a groove in the foam, first methodically with my house keys and, when that wasn't working, frantically with my fingers. Fragments sprayed every-where, leaving white pebbles of foam debris that stayed embedded in the thin, brown office carpet for months. An hour's work later, the syringe fit snugly. The medication, which did not require refrigeration, arrived intact via courier at our contact near the woman's home. Two days later, a midwife administered the medication at the start of S's labor. Her daughter was born healthy and later tested HIV-free. Infant formula and a subsequent dose of Nevirapine for S at six months helped keep the baby that way, preventing her from contracting the disease through breast milk.

The AIDS Law Project and its sister organization, the Treatment Action Campaign, won a landmark courtroom victory in 2002, mandating that the South African government provide Nevirapine to expectant mothers with HIV.[8] When the government still did not comply, we marched on the central business district of Johannesburg and pretended to die in the streets of the capital, Pretoria. My colleagues fearlessly sued multinational companies for the excessive pricing of their lifesaving HIV medications. It was two more years before the South African government began complying with the court order and HIV treatment slowly became more widely available. As late as 2006, South Africa's health minister was still showing up at international AIDS conferences with a government-sponsored display of vegetable remedies for the disease, including garlic, beetroot, and olive oil. It was only when President Mbeki left office in 2008 that government resistance to HIV treatment programs fully subsided.[9]

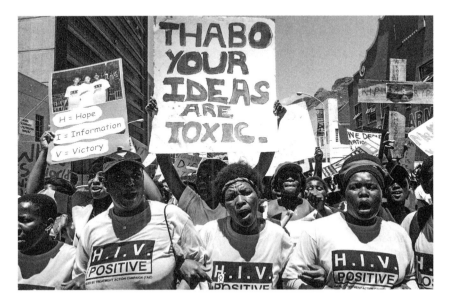

Figure 1.1
AIDS activists protest in Cape Town, South Africa on November 26, 2001.
Photo: Anna Zieminski/AFP/Getty Images.

In the meantime, clients, protest leaders, and good friends of my coworkers had died. Researchers from the Harvard School of Public Health estimated that an additional 35,000 babies were born with HIV and 330,000 people died from AIDS as a result of the South African government's refusal to put in a place a workable treatment and prevention program.[10] That estimate may be conservative; other studies have concluded that the real number of unnecessarily infected infants was nearly twice as high.[11] I worked hard to contribute to the treatment access litigation and protests during my time in South Africa, but when my boss joked that figuring out how to send the syringe would probably be the most useful thing I'd do there, I did not disagree.

I only met S in person once. I told her she had been heroic on behalf of her daughter; she kindly invited me to her wedding. I still think of S and her daughter, who should be 16 years old today.

My time in South Africa occurred at a deeply inequitable moment in global health, especially by historical standards. Although most infectious diseases are now concentrated in tropical and subtropical regions, this is a relatively recent development that dates back only to the start of the twentieth century. Once, plagues and parasites were widespread in the temperate regions of North America, Northern Europe, and East Asia. Yet, by 2003, the share of deaths from infectious diseases in sub-Saharan African countries had become nearly nine times greater than the share in rich nations.[12] That gap is likely the largest geographic disparity in infectious disease in hundreds of years, perhaps even since the end of the Neolithic era when most of humankind had stopped relying on foraging to survive. The way that infectious diseases spread worldwide and then slowly declined in wealthy nations reflects the uneven course of progress in humankind's efforts to overcome the health consequences of its civilizing impulses.

Death, Disease, and the Fall of Prehistoric Man

Infectious diseases are caused by the presence of microorganisms, including viruses, bacteria, mycobacteria, fungi, protozoa, and parasites. Given the heavy presence of these diseases in poorer nations, one might deduce that they are the plagues of less-developed societies. For most of human history, however, the opposite has been true. The burden of infectious diseases grew as humans shifted to farming and villages, domesticated animals, and embraced trade and more rapid transportation, behaviors that are traditionally associated with civilized societies.[13]

Most of what is known about early human encounters with infectious disease comes from archaeological evidence, genetic modeling, and studies of the few hunter-gatherers that continued to exist into the twentieth century. These reconstructions of the history of infectious disease suggest that foragers were poor fodder for most parasites, bacteria, and viruses. Hunter-gatherers traveled in small bands, often numbering thirty to forty people. These foraging bands were mobile and widely scattered, providing few opportunities for disease to spread from person to person. Best estimates are that the average hunter-gatherer needed roughly one square mile to sustain a sufficient diet and moved seven times per year.[14] Many microbes do better indoors, shielded from the disinfecting power of sunlight and the changes in temperature and humidity that came with migration and the search for food.

The infectious diseases that affected early hunter-gatherers came in two varieties. First, there were diseases that arose from occasional encounters with microorganisms that relied primarily on animals for survival (so-called zoonotic diseases). These diseases were deadly because they were unfamiliar to most foragers. Second, there were slow-acting, less fatal diseases, like the bacterial skin disease yaws, that lingered in victims and thereby maximized their chances of being passed to another human host. Rabies and anthrax are examples of the fatal variety of zoonotic diseases believed to have affected hunter-gatherers through incidental contact with infected wild animals. Infection by bacteria, such as tetanus and botulism, and parasites, like trichinosis and other tapeworms, is a risk that comes with butchering and eating wildlife.[15] Diseases carried by flies, mosquitos, rodents, or ticks (vector-borne diseases) probably affected prehistoric societies, but most were limited by geography and climate (bubonic plague was once confined to Egypt and the Great Lakes region of Africa) or were less virulent forms of current diseases (such as the *Plasmodium malariae* and *Plasmodium vivax* forms of malaria).[16] Many of the infectious diseases that became great killers of humankind— such as tuberculosis, pertussis (whooping cough), and typhoid fever—likely loomed at the margins of primitive societies, rising in prominence only when farmers settled down to grow crops, domesticate animals, and live in towns and cities.[17]

The move to villages and farms took hold roughly ten thousand years ago in the Fertile Crescent, a rolling stretch of land that cuts across the

Tigris, Euphrates, and Jordan valleys in modern-day Turkey, Syria, Iran, Iraq, and Israel. Archaeological findings suggest the practice of agriculture arose independently in other regions, and then spread from each of these centers to surrounding communities at varying rates and degrees.[18] By 5000 BCE, the first agrarian villages that relied primarily on planted crops and livestock appeared in the Tigris and Euphrates Valley and domesticated plants were cultivated in the Mediterranean region, China, Pakistan, Central Asia, Peru, Mexico, and the Eastern Sahara. Two thousand years later, all of Europe relied on farming and the practice reached New Guinea. By 1 CE, nearly everyone in the world subsisted on agriculture.[19]

The origins of agriculture are hotly debated, but many scholars now believe that foragers were pushed into agriculture by population pressure, climate change, and droughts rather than drawn by the benefits and charms of farming.[20] The historian Ian Morris speculates that women, who did most of the gathering, are to be thanked, or maybe blamed, for the invention of farming. Men, who did more hunting, were slower (and perhaps lazier) to make a change, but were ultimately responsible for the shift to herding and, eventually, domesticating animals.[21] Both sets of practices had dramatic consequences for infectious disease and human health.

Some consequences of the shift to agriculture were positive. Farming produced more food and bigger populations. Larger and more settled populations could become more acclimated to their environment, which meant greater resilience to the local microbes that still strike international travelers today. A sedentary lifestyle also provided an opportunity to care for the sick. It likewise allowed food storage and the use of heavy ceramic pots, which improved the effectiveness of cooking and likely reduced the incidence of diseases associated with eating raw game and meats.[22]

On balance, however, the toll of infectious disease on human health significantly worsened with agriculture, the domestication of animals, and other advances in civilization.[23] Farming required permanent settlements and yielded larger, more densely populated communities. Archaeological studies of early settlements have found prodigious quantities of discarded refuse, including animal bone scraps, mixed with tool-making debris and human remains.[24] According to the archaeologist Bill Rathje: "Throughout most of time human beings disposed of garbage in a very convenient manner: simply by leaving it where it fell."[25] Unsurprisingly, these permanent settlements attracted vermin, rodents, and insects, and with them came higher rates of deadly infectious diseases, such as yellow fever, toxoplasmosis, and rabies.[26]

Indoor living grouped people closer together without direct sunlight and air circulation to sweep away the bacteria and viruses that cause illnesses like tuberculosis, leprosy, and influenza. Storing food allowed more reliable access to nutrition, but, if not done properly, also gave rise to salmonella, botulism, and other unpleasant bacteria and fungi. With more people comes more waste, human and otherwise. Human waste left to fester in soil can lead to hookworm, an intestinal parasite that troubled the Southeastern United States until 1910 and is still a concern in rural areas of many poor nations today.[27] Waste can also seep into water, breeding bacteria and protozoa that can result in diarrheal diseases, like cholera. Flatworms and flukes thrive in wastewater too and can cause schistosomiasis, an ancient parasitic disease that can lead to kidney failure, liver damage, and death.[28]

The domestication of animals increased their size, herded them together, and brought them into closer contact with people.[29] A murderers' row of infectious diseases are believed to have arisen or intensified as a result. Measles, diphtheria, and rotavirus (a diarrheal disease) originated from cattle, goats, and sheep; influenza and trichinosis from pigs and poultry; and the common cold from camels.[30] The exchange of diseases also went the other way; recent genomic research suggests humans are responsible for tapeworms and tuberculosis in cows.[31]

Farming and irrigation are also labor intensive, requiring the presence of lots of workers and cattle for plowing, and these activities produce ditches that collect rainwater—an ideal setting for mosquitos to breed and spread malaria.[32] Clearing the equatorial forests in Africa for farms is thought to have led to the development of a strain of malaria, *Plasmodium falciparum*, that may have killed more people than any other infectious disease.[33] The clearing of land for cultivation may have also disrupted the habitats of rodents and wildlife, increasing the chance of transmission of new and existing diseases to villagers and farm workers, such as smallpox and bubonic plague.[34]

One measure of the increased burden of infectious disease that came with the adoption of agriculture, animal domestication, and other civilized lifestyles is that, despite more reliable access to food, there is no evidence of any sustained increase in life expectancy for thousands of years after the shift to agriculture in any region of the world. Studies of skeletal remains in Iran, Iraq, and the Midwestern United States from before and after the transition to agriculture suggest that rates of viral and bacterial infections worsened. Women in these early agricultural societies could expect to have four to seven births during their reproductive lives, but lost more than a

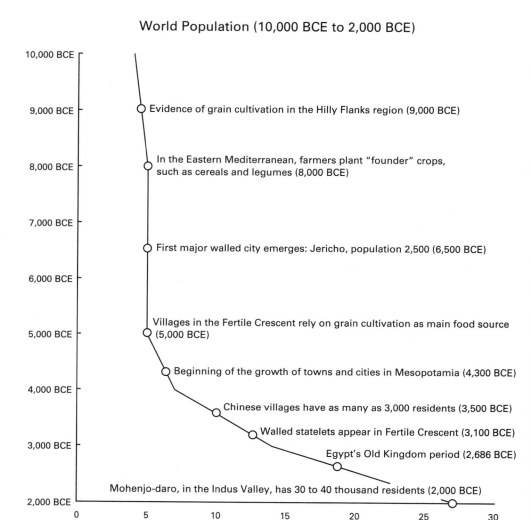

Figure 1.2
Sources: McEvedy and Jones, *Atlas of World Population History*, 1978; Kremer,
"Population Growth and Technological Change," 1993; Williams, *Cassell's Chronology
of World History* 2005; Scott, *Against the Grain*, 2017; Bairoch, *Cities and Economic
Development*, 1988; Morris, *Why the West Rules*, 2010.

third of their children before their fifth birthdays, a higher rate than is estimated for their foraging predecessors. Childbirth was a dominant cause of death for these women. Even with increased fertility, the population of early agricultural societies grew steadily but slowly, until around 3000 BCE and the emergence of the first states.[35]

The earliest states were walled cities in southern Mesopotamia, Egypt, the Indus Valley, and the Yellow River basin, which began to exhibit an appreciable division of labor and developed an apparatus for exerting social, political, and economic control over their residents. As the political scientist James C. Scott has observed, these first footholds of civilization were all agrarian and founded in flat, alluvial plains; all were grain-based societies. To function, these states had to maintain a sufficient number of laborers to do the drudgery of producing the agricultural surpluses and wool textiles needed to support elites and the other members of the hierarchical social order (priests, clerks, soldiers, artisans). Wars of this era tended not to be over territory, but instead amounted to military raids to seize people and plunder from nearby foraging bands and smaller settlements.[36]

These early states emerged in silted floodplains with plentiful water and rich soil that were great for growing grain, fishing, and grazing livestock, but lacked the commodities that the new elites coveted and the strategic necessities for state-building. The Sumerian city-state of Uruk (in what is now southern Iraq) established the first trade network to exchange barley, textiles, and dates for copper and obsidian (black volcanic rock) for weapons and tools, timber and limestone for building, and ivory for art.[37] The advent of coastal sailing vessels enabled longer-distance commerce, faster travel, and more regular contact with other human settlements. Ancient Egypt had Red Sea trade routes that extended 1,500 miles into present-day Yemen. By 400 BCE, Phoenician and Greek traders roamed throughout the Mediterranean and Black Sea, up and down the eastern and western African coasts, and eventually reached India. Centuries later, the Roman Empire extended these arteries of commerce, shipping tin from Cornwall, wines from Tuscany, and a lot of silver to buy the Chinese silks, pepper from the Malabar Coast, and exotic wildlife pets from India that wealthy Romans craved.[38]

Urban centers, seafaring trade, and military might fueled the greatness and glory of Rome and other early civilizations, but the epidemiological consequences were staggering. According to Scott, the first states in Mesopotamia "represented a ten- to twentyfold increase in population density over anything Homo sapiens had ever experienced."[39] The population of Babylon, the first great city of antiquity, was between 200,000 and 300,000. Athens had roughly a hundred thousand residents at its peak. Rome was home to one million people by the late first century BCE and was surrounded by a galaxy of smaller cities.[40] These settlements and walled city-states, packed with people, rodents, and livestock, were feedlots for the germs and parasites that accompanied marching armies, trade caravans, and questionable personal hygiene.

Diseases resembling tuberculosis, typhus, bubonic plague, smallpox, and leprosy appear in early Sumerian writings as far back as 2000 BCE.[41] In the book of Deuteronomy in the Old Testament, written around 700 BCE, God promises the Hebrews that a return to their sparsely populated homeland from the congested cities of Egypt will "take away all the sickness from…the foul diseases of Egypt which you know so well."[42] Dysentery, typhoid, and other food- and fecal-borne infectious diseases were likely the great, everyday killers of early urban living, but it is the epidemics that history remembers.[43] Thucydides describes a plague in the second year of the Peloponnesian War that arrived in the port of Piraeus via Egypt and Libya, killed one-fourth of the army and innumerable residents, and left Athens in a "state of unprecedented lawlessness."[44] Marcus Aurelius and his legions brought back from Mesopotamia in 165 CE a still-unidentified infection, known as the Antonine Plague, which caused the deaths of a third of Rome's residents, including Aurelius's co-Emperor.[45] Surges of infectious disease repeatedly battered and depopulated the Roman Empire in the subsequent decades until it was overrun by nomadic tribes.[46] In 541 CE, the Plague of Justinian, now believed to be bubonic plague, spread along maritime supply lines across Egypt into Constantinople.[47] It ravaged the Mediterranean world in eighteen waves, with an average of one epidemic every twelve years. The population of Rome fell to 20,000. By the end of the seventh century, the combination of recurrent attacks of plague and constant war had halved the population of Europe and hastened the collapse of the Byzantine Empire.[48] The same disease arrived at China's seaports in 610 and did its worst damage in the populated south and coastal provinces. The weakened Tang dynasty lost control over the Silk Road, and trade between Europe and Asia virtually disappeared.[49]

The era that followed is known as the Dark Ages, when Europe receded into a poor agricultural society with few large towns or cities and little written record, but health actually improved during this time. Agriculture thrived amid warm, stable climatic conditions. For six centuries, there was little contact between Europe and Asia, and their disease pools were kept largely separate.

Between 1000 and 1300, Europe's population doubled to its largest size in a thousand years. New walled cities were founded and became more densely populated, with as many as 100,000 residents. Europe's population grew from 26 million inhabitants in the eighth century to 80 million at the start of the fourteenth century. By some estimates, the population of Asia at that time was as much as five times larger. The roads left in ruins since the fall of Rome were rebuilt. The Mongol conquests cleared and reopened the Silk Road to overland trade. The Mediterranean maritime trading network reemerged, and improvements in boat design allowed swifter, year-round shipping, which had been impossible centuries earlier.[50]

With population growth and burgeoning trade between settlements, epidemics of infectious disease resurged, crashing against Europe in deadly waves starting in the 1330s. A plague, which later became known as the Black Death, emerged out of Central Asia. The exact origin of the epidemic in Europe is uncertain, but some historians have attributed its start to the Tartar siege of a Genoese trading outpost in Caffa (now Feodosia, Ukraine) in 1346, where the attackers may have passed the disease on to the defenders by flinging infected corpses over the city walls with a catapult.[51] Once the epidemic began, however, there is no question that it spread along both maritime and the overland Silk Road trading routes.[52]

For seven years, the Black Death ravaged Europe, Central Asia, and North Africa. Unlike most epidemic infections, transmission depended less on the crowding of people and more on the density of the colonies of rats and their fleas that spread the disease, and so the Black Death struck cities and villages alike.[53] One survivor described bodies laid in mass graves in Florence in layers of dirt "just as one makes lasagna with layers of pasta and cheese."[54] A father's account from Siena describes burying his five children with his own hands and so many dying that "all believed it was the end of the world."[55] By 1353, an estimated one-third of all Europeans had died from the plague—roughly 25 million out of a population of 75 million perished in under a decade.[56] The plague made frequent returns over the next several centuries and the continent's population did not fully recover for nearly three hundred years. The loss of life in the Islamic world may have

The Spread of Black Death along Land and Sea Trade Routes, 1346 to 1353

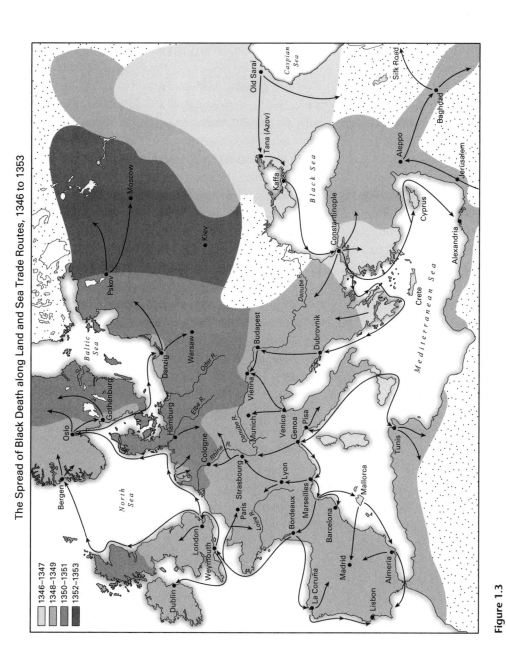

Figure 1.3

Adapted from Benedictow, *The Black Death 1346–1353* (2006).

been even more severe.[57] The Asyut region of Egypt lost 98 percent of its taxpayers and the roads from Cairo to Palestine were littered with corpses.[58] The great Arab historian Ibn Khaldun lost both of his parents when the Black Death swept through Tunis. Years later, he wrote:

> Civilization both in the East and the West was visited by a destructive plague which devastated nations and caused populations to vanish. It swallowed up many of the good things of civilization and wiped them out.[59]

While there is no doubt that the Black Death plague led to dramatic shifts in civilization in Europe and the affected parts of Asia and Africa, not all those changes were bad. With the collapse of population in Europe, for instance, labor became scarce. This led to an increase in wages and living standards, especially in Northern Europe, and the collapse of the feudal system.[60] There were greater investments in labor-saving inventions, such as the printing press.[61] Capitalism began to flourish, land was better distributed, and power became more centralized in the nation-state. With more administrative power and a greater ability to tax and raise revenues, rulers could fund commercial expeditions and exploration.[62] Yet, with these advances in civilization, the threat of infectious disease only grew greater and more widespread.

Before Christopher Columbus landed on the shores of the Bahamas, smallpox, measles, cholera, influenza, and many other infectious diseases did not exist in the Americas.[63] The Native American populations that resided in the New World at that time had descended from migrants who crossed over the Siberian land bridge from Northern Asia thousands of years earlier and remained relatively isolated. Few animals were domesticated in the region, and those that were did not match up to the cows, pigs, and horses of Europe and Asia as good incubators of disease. Muscovy ducks, turkeys, and llamas do not live in large flocks or herds, were not kept indoors or in large numbers, and people do not drink their milk.[64]

The historical isolation of Native American populations and their limited exposure to disease-ridden cattle matters because the human immune system develops through exposure to disease. Each new invading pathogen produces long-lasting memory cells that allow survivors to mount a robust response should that same pathogen reappear. Without that prior exposure to many infectious diseases, the indigenous populations of the Americas and the other more remote continents of the world were wiped out in large part by the viruses, bacteria, and parasites that accompanied European exploration, colonization, and conquest.[65]

Within two hundred years, three-quarters of the native population of the Americas would disappear, mostly as a result of infectious disease. Historian William McNeill identified smallpox and measles as the reasons why, in 1521, Hernán Cortés, with fewer than six hundred men, was able to conquer the Aztec Empire, which numbered in the millions. McNeill wrote:

> Whenever a new region or hitherto isolated Amerindian population came into regular contact with the outside world, the cycle of repeated infections picked up renewed force, mowing down the helpless inhabitants.[66]

Around three million Aztecs in Mexico died of smallpox, measles, and a dozen other infectious diseases that had not been previously introduced to the region.[67] A Spanish friar described the Aztecs dying "in heaps, like bedbugs … because, as they were all taken sick at once, they could not care for each other."[68] A similar fate would befall the Inca Empire and its 80,000-strong army, which Francisco Pizarro managed to subdue in 1532 with a force of 168 men, only 62 of whom had horses.[69] After Columbus's arrival on the island of Hispaniola, a combination of outbreaks of smallpox and other infections nearly extinguished the indigenous population.[70]

By the time the Pilgrims arrived, as many as 90 percent of the Native Americans who had been living in New England had already perished from smallpox and other infectious diseases that explorers and earlier would-be settlers brought with them.[71] Violence, forced displacement, and subjugation had created ideal conditions for the spread of infectious diseases, crowding Native Americans together in stressful circumstances without sufficient food or sanitation.[72] The Europeans took the plight of the Native Americans as God's blessing to take their land. John Winthrop, the first governor of Massachusetts, wrote: "The natives, they are neere all dead of the small Poxe, so as the Lord hathe cleared our title to what we possess."[73] In some instances, the colonists helped the Lord remove the cloud over their title to the land by distributing blankets from smallpox patients to surrounding Native American tribes, an early form of biological warfare.[74]

The steep decline in the indigenous American population spurred European involvement in the West African slave trade, which Arab traders had been operating at a much smaller scale. The slave trade brought yellow fever and the deadly malaria parasite *Plasmodium falciparum* to the Caribbean, South America, and the southeastern United States. Malariologist

Marshall A. Barber summed up the link between the spread of malaria and slavery as "the Dark Continent aveng[ing] itself for the theft of its children."[75] High rates of malaria in these regions were sustained by the conditions at sugar and cotton plantations, which were poorly drained, housed livestock, and "employed" thousands of undernourished plantation workers—a perfect environment for mosquitos.[76] Yellow fever, even more lethal, spread with the *Aedes aegypti* mosquito that favors the water casks on trading ships and rain-filled barrels and cisterns in urban areas.[77] Some believe that one infectious disease—syphilis—originated in the Americas and was brought by the explorers and the conquistadors back to Europe, but this question remains unsettled.[78]

What is more certain is that after the Age of Exploration and the expansion of the slave trade, the incidence and variety of infectious disease differed by geography and ecosystem (more in tropics and less in deserts and frozen tundra), but much less so than now or over the last couple of centuries.[79] With the increase of trade that came with the discovery of maritime routes to Asia and the Americas, a new network of commercial cities arose in Northern Europe. This network started with cities like Lisbon, Bruges, and Antwerp and later expanded to Amsterdam and London.[80] To the extent that there were differences in the global toll of infectious disease, that toll was likely worse in these more economically developed and densely populated societies.[81] As the anthropologist Mark Nathan Cohen has written:

> A good case can be made that the urban populations of Europe [in the fourteenth and eighteenth centuries] may have been the most nutritionally impoverished, disease-ridden, and shortest-lived populations in human history....Modern civilizations are clearly successful in the sense that they provide for increasing numbers of people, even if they have added little to the health and nutrition of the individuals until quite recently.[82]

It is tempting to see the adoption of farming, pastoralism, permanent settlements, and trade as humankind's fall from grace, from foraging the Garden of Eden to subsisting in the drudgery of sedentary, agricultural life and the grip of death and infectious disease. This is, after all, the view put forward in the book of Genesis, where God casts out Adam and Eve for having eaten the fruit of knowledge and condemns the couple and their descendants to a life of farming:

> I have placed a curse on the ground. All your life you will struggle to scratch a living from it. It will grow thorns and thistles for you, though you will eat of its grains. All your life you will sweat to produce food, until your dying day.[83]

The anthropologist and Pulitzer Prize winner Jared Diamond agrees with that dim assessment, calling agriculture the "worst mistake in the history of the human race," which led to shorter lives, tyranny, and war.[84]

It is hard to disagree with the Bible and Jared Diamond, but their fondness for foraging may be overstated. Steven Pinker's book *Better Angels of Our Nature* summarizes the extensive research that shows that many hunter-gatherer societies were deeply violent. War accounted for a staggering share of deaths, as many as half in some cases, and there is evidence of widespread cannibalism.[85]

What is undeniable is that a great project of humankind over the past several millennia has been striving to overcome the health consequences of our civilizing choices. That project has been global and, for most of human history, spectacularly unsuccessful. Population growth was cyclical, interrupted by famine, pestilence, and war, with only small gains occurring over very long periods. Estimates of the average life expectancy (25 years) in Britain in 1728 are not much better than those for Rome at the height of its empire (22 years) or ancient Greece (18 years).[86] Until a couple of hundred years ago, lives were short and health conditions miserable, with high death rates, high birth rates, and a heavy burden of infectious disease more or less everywhere.

The Path to Better Health in Wealthier Nations

Health conditions began to improve slowly around 1650, starting in Britain, Sweden, and Northern Europe and later spreading to societies with deep European roots such as the United States, New Zealand, and Australia. The health gains in these nations started well before the discovery of effective medical treatments.[87] The first vaccine was invented in 1796. Sulfonamide-based medicines ("sulfa drugs"), penicillin, and other antibiotics did not appear until the 1920s and 1930s. Many have rightly cited improved nutrition and the rise in incomes that came with the Industrial Revolution as playing a role in these early health gains, although researchers and historians still debate their relative contributions.[88] Economist and Nobel Laureate Angus Deaton points out that, until 1750, gains in life expectancy for the well-fed and wealthy British nobility were no better than for the general population.[89] The residents of the rising industrial cities in Europe were better paid than their rural counterparts, but health in these smoke-choked urban centers was much worse. The average life expectancy of the inhabitants of Liverpool and Manchester in 1841 was more than a decade lower than those living in the British countryside.[90] Better-nourished children were less likely to die and better able to ward off disease, but the infants who did not benefit directly from improvements in nutrition also enjoyed better survival rates.[91] Changes in social norms, advances in the understanding of infectious disease, and more responsive government were also important drivers of progress.

In the seventeenth and eighteenth centuries, the prevailing social attitude toward the poor and children ranged from indifferent to hostile. Reverend Thomas Robert Malthus published his *Essay on the Principle of Population* in 1798, arguing that "except in extreme cases, the actual progress of population is little affected by unhealthiness or healthiness" and that improving their condition would only risk exhausting the food supply and wider famine.[92] Those who take their children to see a performance of *A Christmas Carol*, as I did this year, will hear Charles Dickens depicting this prevailing attitude through the words of his protagonist Ebenezer Scrooge:

> "Since you ask me what I wish, gentlemen, that is my answer. I don't make merry myself at Christmas and I can't afford to make idle people merry. I help support the establishments I have mentioned: they cost enough and those who are badly off must go there." "Many can't go there; and many would rather die." "If they would rather die," said Scrooge, "they have better do it, and decrease the surplus population."[93]

Changes in this attitude began with the Enlightenment. The writings of the English philosopher Jeremy Bentham were influential, arguing that the objectives of society should be the "greatest happiness of the greatest number." That utilitarian notion helped inspire social reformers to press for improved sanitation in Europe's fast-growing cities.[94] A new view of infancy as a time of uncorrupted goodness spurred a social movement in France for women to breastfeed and ensure the cleanliness of their children.[95] Similar efforts followed in Britain with lectures, penny pamphlets, and volunteer initiatives, like the Ladies' National Association for the Diffusion of Sanitary Knowledge.[96] Efforts to control the number of births started in France and were initially achieved through withdrawal or abstinence. Evangelical Christians, who followed a gospel of social action exemplified by the writings of Charles Dickens, opened general hospitals and dispensaries and provided free care to children and the "deserving poor."[97] Private philanthropists funded and promoted inoculation from smallpox, a disease that still caused 10 percent of all deaths in Europe at that time.[98] Greater appreciation of population growth as a means of expanding foreign empires, armies, and national economic growth led some European governments to invest in infant survival and motherhood education programs as "matter[s] of Imperial importance."[99]

This combination of movements improved social norms and hygiene in Northern Europe, helping reduce the death toll of infectious disease and infant deaths. It also marked the start of an unlikely coalition of nationalists, philanthropists, secular social reformers, and evangelical Christians that would reemerge centuries later in the fight against the HIV/AIDS epidemic in sub-Saharan Africa. A straight line, for instance, may be drawn from the Benthamite message that "all human beings have a natural capacity to earn a living and learn, and ought not to be prevented from doing so by illness or untimely death" and the motto of the Bill and Melinda Gates Foundation: "All people should have the opportunity to lead healthy, productive lives."[100]

Despite the progress made by these early social reformers, most of Europe remained regularly battered by epidemics of cholera, dysentery, typhus, and typhoid. Chapter 4 discusses these urban diseases at greater length. For now, suffice to say, these diseases killed in far lesser numbers than the plagues of medieval Europe but still inspired great terror. In the nineteenth century, riots broke out in response to epidemics of cholera in cities across Eastern and Western Europe, Russia, and North and South America. These riots were not coordinated and occurred in strikingly different economies and political systems. In Liverpool and New York City, rioters attacked medical professionals and hospitals. In Hungary, castles were attacked and nobles murdered. In Naples, mobs attacked the offices of the national government over its incompetence in improving the city's sanitary conditions and infrastructure after years of false promises.[101]

The priority for governments and elites became being seen to do something in response to cholera, to implement any policy in which the confidence of the public might be maintained or restored. At first, many of the actions undertaken were ineffective or even counterproductive.[102] But the terror of infectious disease continued to spur action amid a rising middle class and a new generation of social reformers and physicians who were less likely to defer to divine intervention or be satisfied with ineffective remedies. Their actions led to two developments that dramatically accelerated the decline of infectious diseases and extended progress beyond a handful of European nations.[103]

The first development was a cluster of discoveries that yielded the germ theory of disease. The prevailing view in the early nineteenth century had been that disease stemmed from the loose morals of its sufferers and poisonous gases emanating from dirty environments and standing water. Avoiding foul water and disposing of waste do reduce the chances of getting sick, but this notion of disease as filth also led to crackdowns against immigrants, prostitutes, and religious minorities and overlooked microbial threats that could not be easily perceived by sight or smell. The first blow struck against this view of disease was physician John Snow's classic 1854 study that identified a water pump on Broad Street in London as the source of contaminated water that spread cholera. The subsequent discoveries of Robert Koch, Joseph Lister, and Louis Pasteur provided the scientific basis for Snow's observation, establishing microbes, not merely bad smells or poor morals, as the agents of disease. Collectively, these discoveries established the new fields of epidemiology and microbiology and led to the identification of the causative microorganisms for tuberculosis, cholera, and typhoid, and many other infectious diseases. Equally important, germ theory contributed to a second critical development: the emergence of public health systems to put these ideas into practice for the public good.

To be effective, germ theory needed to be paired with governments able to act in response to the health and social concerns of its citizens. This was a more revolutionary development than it sounds. Outbreaks of cholera and yellow fever led to the establishment of the first municipal health boards and public health laws in London and many other European and American cities.[104] Under pressure from angry citizens, social reformers, and industry, city governments in other European nations also began building systems to distribute water and evacuate liquid waste. The adoption of sanitation was so rapid in Europe that it became known as "water mania."[105] Sanitation and safer water systems in many US cities required a longer fight. Americans were more fearful of government paternalism and often favored private contractors to provide basic city services such as street cleaning and clean water. Nepotism and corruption were rampant in many US city governments, and contractors cut corners and frequently abandoned service amid epidemics. After decades of scandals and social mobilization for greater political reform, US municipal governments began to assume more responsibility for the construction of sewers and aqueducts. By the start of the twentieth century, there were nearly 1,700 public water systems in the United States, and city governments spent more on them than the federal government devoted to anything other than the postal service and the military.[106]

The public health bodies required to establish and maintain effective sanitation systems have continued to drive reductions in infectious disease and change the role of government in the daily lives of people. They later passed laws to close down tenements, which cut rates of tuberculosis, and to require the pasteurization of milk. David Cutler and Grant Miller estimate that 43 percent of the decline in mortality in US cities between 1900 and 1936 can be attributed to water filtration and chlorination.[107] From 1850 to 1920, the combination of these public health efforts dramatically cut infant mortality in the wealthier nations of Europe, countries with strong European roots (Australia, Canada, New Zealand, and the United States), and Japan to levels that many lower-income nations have reached only recently.[108]

In sum, most of the reduction in infectious diseases and improvements in health in these first-mover nations were achieved at fairly low levels of technological sophistication. They were the products of changing social norms and education, a better understanding of the causes of disease, and the development of public health institutions and responsive governance to implement that knowledge. Wealth alone did not ensure reduction in infectious disease. In some industrializing nations, declining mortality rates predated the long climb to improved living standards.[109]

The historian Mark Harrison has argued that infectious diseases created the conditions in which the modern state and the machinery of government emerged.[110] Meeting the threat of plagues and parasites required coordinated government action and the advancement of the public good over countervailing commercial and individual interests. The specific actions undertaken varied, depending on that country's prior experience with epidemic threats and the administrative capacity and resources of the government.[111] But the types of measures undertaken—quarantine, vaccination, housing reforms, and sanitation and safe water systems—set the precedent for other forms of social regulation, such as compulsory schooling, improved public administration, and investment in urban infrastructure.[112]

This was not, however, an experience shared by all nations. Impoverished countries disrupted by colonialism had little opportunity to build sewers and safe water systems, or to put the lessons of germ theory to good

Is Your City in the Vanguard Fighting Water-Borne Typhoid?

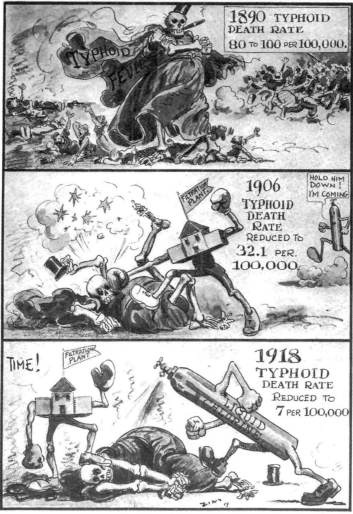

Cartoon drawn specially for THE AMERICAN CITY *by Zim*

Figure 1.4
Cartoon by Eugene "Zim" Zimmerman, *American City* 21 (Sept. 1919): 247.

use. Colonial powers determined how and where to invest in responding to the disease threats, and they generally favored their own protection over sustainable, systemic public health investments in their colonies.[113] Colonialism not only stripped countries of resources and impeded political development; it left local elites less accountable to their citizens. After independence, many nations were left with predatory rulers. A collapse of world commodity prices in the 1970s and the debt crisis that ensued in the 1980s forced many countries, particularly in Latin America and sub-Saharan Africa, to drastically cut government support for health-care systems and social services, sometimes under pressure from their lenders, the World Bank and International Monetary Fund.[114]

The health differences between "have" and "have-not" nations have only grown with the discovery and development of better medical tools.[115] Sulfa drugs emerged from the dye industry in the 1930s and were the first effective treatments for many bacterial infections.[116] Penicillin and other antibiotics followed a decade later. New antitoxins and vaccines were developed for tetanus and diphtheria (1890), whooping cough (1914), yellow fever (1936), influenza (1943), polio (1955), measles (1963), mumps (1967), rubella (1969), and hepatitis B (1981). The development of antiretroviral medicines changed the course of the HIV/AIDS epidemic, which gained prominence first in the United States and Europe in the 1980s before disproportionately affecting poor countries, especially in sub-Saharan Africa. The development of these medical technologies and the high cost and inaccessibility of some of them, especially drugs for HIV/AIDS, contributed to the great global inequity in health and infectious disease that characterized the time when I was living in South Africa.

A Better World Begins as a More Unequal One

Angus Deaton has argued that in the history of human health, rarely has progress been equally distributed; the path to a better world usually starts with a more unequal one.

We have few country-level data to assess that claim and the course of long-term progress in human health and infectious disease. Many readers of this book may take it for granted that they have a birth certificate, and that when they die, their death and its cause will be officially recorded. Yet, in more than one hundred nations, and not just the most destitute ones, these basic birth and death registration systems are lacking. Even fewer countries produce decent vital statistics, which depend on doctors correctly assigning the cause of death.[117] More reliable, country-level estimates on the global causes of death and infirmity date back only to 1990 and are the product of the Global Burden of Disease project, a groundbreaking effort run by Christopher Murray at the University of Washington that involves thousands of researchers worldwide.

One of the few longer-run measures of the health of a country's population is estimated average life expectancy at birth. It is an imprecise measure of health and an even less reliable means of evaluating changes in the toll and incidence of infectious disease. But it is the best long-run measure we have and it offers some insights. Life expectancy is sensitive to changes in infant and child mortality (people dying at age one affect the average more than people perishing at age thirty), and many of the causes of infant and child deaths have historically been infections.

Figure 1.5 is adapted from the Our World in Data project at the University of Oxford, led by economist Max Roser, and uses data from the Gapminder

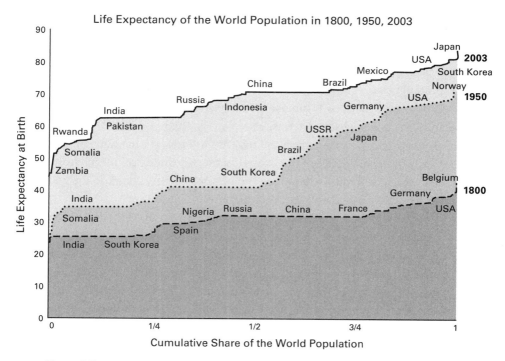

Figure 1.5
Adapted from Max Roser/Our World in Data. Data source: Gapminder.

Foundation.[118] This figure shows the average life expectancy of the world population at various points in history, with annotations indicating the share of population that comes from particular countries. In 1800 (the dashed line), no country had an average life expectancy above 40 and no nation had an average life expectancy below 25, a fairly narrow band. By 1950 (the dotted line), nations in Europe and North America had experienced dramatic improvements in life expectancy, reaching as high as 71 years. This progress occurred even though effective medical treatments, such as penicillin, had become available only very recently and many of today's most important vaccines, such as for polio or measles, had not yet been developed. On the other hand, life expectancy in many nations, such as India, had hardly advanced at all, with a life expectancy of 34 years. The gap between the countries with the best and worst life expectancy was 38 years.

By 2003 (the solid line), which is shortly after I left South Africa, infectious disease played only a small role in the health of wealthy nations. Life expectancy at birth exceeded 80 years, on average, in countries such as Japan, Iceland, Australia, and Italy. China, Brazil, Indonesia, and India—populous developing nations—had also dramatically lifted the health of their citizens, with improved life expectancies ranging from 63 to 72 years. Yet, in other lower-income countries in sub-Saharan Africa such as Zimbabwe, Swaziland, and Zambia, in the midst of a raging HIV/AIDS epidemic, life expectancy was as low as 44. That gap in longevity between the poorest and wealthiest nations is almost certainly the largest in recorded human history, at least in absolute terms.

That is a shocking statistic, but it may be outdone by what happens next. After 2003, the incidence of infectious disease decreased not just in wealthy countries and emerging economies, but in sub-Saharan Africa and the poorest parts of South Asia as well, as can be seen in figure 1.6.

How were these long-awaited reductions in infectious disease achieved? Not in the same ways as they had been in wealthy nations or even in countries like China. Improvements in education and social norms, especially around breastfeeding and childbirth, have played a similar salutary role in poorer nations as they did in wealthy ones. Yet, the recent gains in health have happened in many countries without the better public health institutions, more responsive governance, and the same improvement in living standards that characterized wealthy nations' escape from infectious disease.[119]

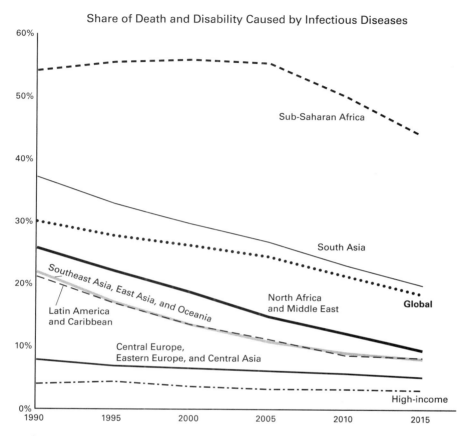

Figure 1.6
Data source: Institute for Health Metrics and Evaluation, Global Burden of Disease (GBD), 2015.

The key to this recent progress appears to have been international donors, intergovernmental agencies, and local governments finding a solution to the same problem that S faced in South Africa. They too found a way to get lifesaving medicines to the world's poorest people, still firmly in the deadly grasp of infectious disease. The HIV/AIDS epidemic in South Africa and other nations accelerated this international effort, but the strategy used to do it has its roots in colonial and military health. The next chapter tells that story.

2   Diseases of Conquest and Colony

Humanity does not have to live in a world of plagues, disastrous governments, conflict, and uncontrolled health risks. The coordinated action of a group of dedicated people can plan for and bring about a better future. The fact of smallpox eradication remains a constant reminder that we should settle for nothing less.

—William H. Foege, *House on Fire*[1]

If you are over 30 and not from Ethiopia, it may be impossible to think of that country without images of children starving. In October 1984, BBC broadcast news of a famine occurring amid a long, bitter civil war in the Tigray province in the Northern Highlands. The Derg, the military dictatorship in power, had withheld food aid and used the famine to push rural residents into camps to deprive the rebels of their supporters. The images from those camps were appalling: listless, emaciated girls and boys in dusty camps with bellies protruding, flies crawling across their faces and eyes. A half of a million people died in the famine. The footage inspired efforts to raise relief funds, including a Christmas song by British pop stars ("Do They Know It's Christmas?"), another song by international recording artists ("We Are the World"), and simultaneous live concerts in London and Philadelphia. My sister had the 45 record of the British single and my siblings and I sang our off-key inquiries after Africans' cognizance of Christmas for months. (As it happens, most Ethiopians are Christians and were likely aware of the holiday.)[2] Footage of Ethiopia's famine featured in NGO fundraising ads for years. Development economists Abhijit Banerjee and Esther Duflo have said that "no single event affecting the world's poor has captured the public imagination and prompted collective generosity as much as the Ethiopian famine of the early 1980's."[3]

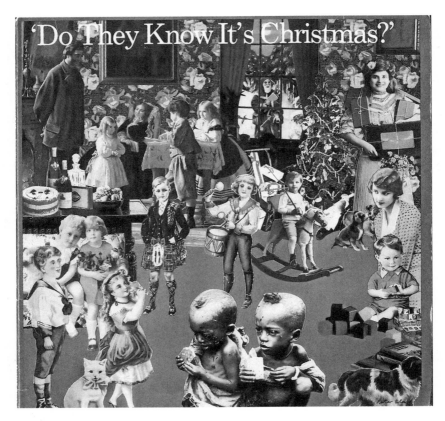

Figure 2.1
UK supergroup Band Aid, Columbia Records (1984). Image courtesy of Andrea
Bollyky Purcell, published pursuant to fair use.

Today, the health and nutrition of most Ethiopians is much improved.
Malaria, HIV, tuberculosis, and most other infectious diseases have
declined. Premature deaths from malaria alone fell by a whopping 96 percent since 2005.[4] Those improvements have contributed to the two-thirds
decline in infant mortality in Ethiopia since 1990. With fewer children
dying, families and governments are making greater investments in education. Enrollment of primary-school-age children in Ethiopia went from
22 percent in 1995 to 74 percent in 2010. The average Ethiopian woman
now gives birth to four children instead of eight.[5] Ethiopia is one of
just eight countries worldwide where the life expectancy of women has
improved by ten or more years in the short span of a single decade. The

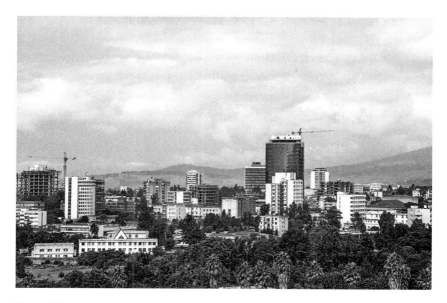

Figure 2.2
The skyline of the downtown business district in Addis Ababa, Ethiopia, 2015.
Photo: Getty Images.

eight-year gains in Ethiopian men's life spans over that time are nearly as impressive.[6]

With improved health, the population in Ethiopia is growing fast, swelling from 48 million in 1990 to 104 million people in 2017, and the economy is keeping pace.[7] Ethiopia is one of the world's most rapidly growing economies over the last five years, according to the International Monetary Fund. Nearly every street in central Addis Ababa, the country's capital, seems to feature a high-rise under construction. Having traveled to Ethiopia for work over the years, I find it hard to come away unimpressed by the transformation. One measure of global esteem for the great health advances made in Ethiopia came with the election of Tedros Adhanom Ghebreyesus, the country's former health minister, to lead the World Health Organization—the first African to ever hold that post.

The recent progress against plagues and parasites is not limited to Ethiopia. The rates of infectious diseases are falling dramatically everywhere, even in developing countries where the economy is not growing as fast as Ethiopia's. The following data and figures come from the Global Burden of

Disease project at the University of Washington and highlight these positive trends.[8]

Malaria deaths worldwide decreased by nearly 27 percent from their peak in 2003, when that disease annually claimed roughly one million lives. Deaths from HIV/AIDS globally have fallen from 1.9 million in 2005 to 1.1 million. Tuberculosis, which once killed 80 percent of those infected in nineteenth-century Europe, now takes about a quarter fewer lives than it did just a decade ago. Deaths from diarrheal diseases, a terrible killer of children in poor countries, have also fallen by more than a fifth over the same period. Measles, the disease that once ravaged the Inca and Roman empires, causes one-quarter of the deaths (68,220) that it did just a decade ago.

Deaths from most of the exotic parasites, bacterial blights, and obscure viruses that are largely confined to the poorest countries in tropical regions are also down sharply.[9] Rabies and leishmaniasis each kill half as many people as a decade ago. The death toll of African trypanosomiasis, a parasitic disease also known as sleeping sickness, has decreased by more than three-quarters. The list goes on. As figure 2.3 shows, there has been an across-the-board

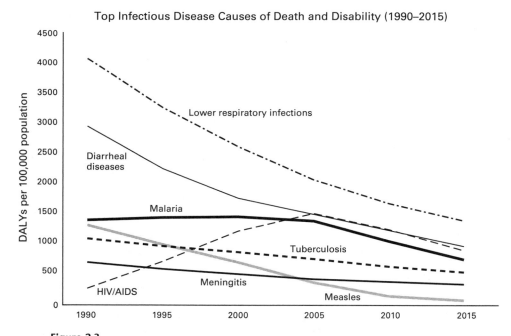

Figure 2.3
Data source: Institute for Health Metrics and Evaluation, GBD 2015.

global decline in the death and disability caused by all of the major infectious diseases (as measured here in disability-adjusted life years or DALYs).

The progress in reducing infectious diseases has reverberated through the other traditional measures of health. In 1960, nearly one in four children born in developing countries died before his or her fifth birthday. The rates in sub-Saharan Africa were even higher.[10] As a result of the improvements in health, there has been a staggering 78 percent decline in child mortality in lower-income countries over the last fifty-five years. The rate of child death has decreased in every single developing country in the world. There are no exceptions. Figure 2.4 shows the drop in child mortality by geographic region. The progress has been spectacular.

As the mortality rates of children have fallen, so has the need for women in lower-income nations to have so many of them. In the early 1960s, women in developing countries gave birth to six children, on average, over the course of their lives. By 2010, that rate had plunged to roughly three

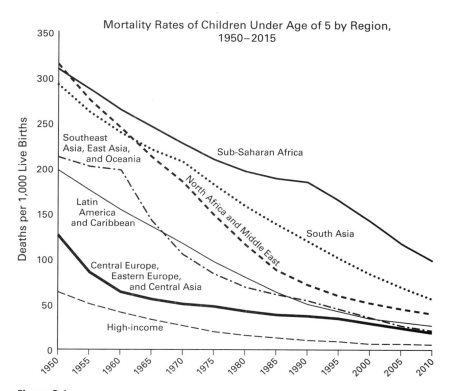

Figure 2.4
Data source: UN Population Prospects.

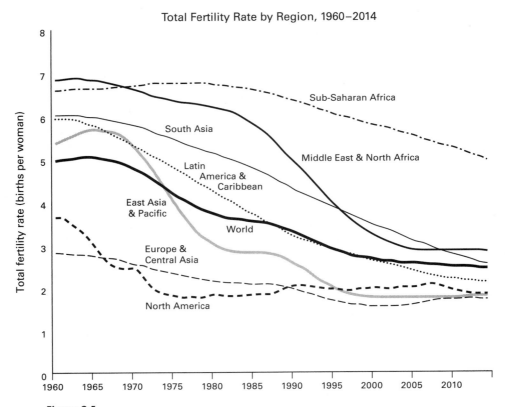

Figure 2.5
Data source: World Bank, World Development Indicators.

children, although, as figure 2.5 shows, the pace of decline has been slower in sub-Saharan Africa. Fertility rates are important because childbirth affects women's health, especially in nations with poor health care, and having too many children too early can keep women from getting an education and entering the workforce. The declining birth rates in lower-income countries have helped reduce the annual number of maternal deaths, which has fallen by 230,000 since 1990. The lives of several million women in poor nations have been saved over the last twenty-five years.

The dramatic gains in health have led to stunning improvements in the average life expectancy of people born in developing nations. In 1990, a newborn in a low-income country could expect to live to be 53 years old. By 2015, that metric had improved to 62 years. In those twenty-five years, the gap between the life expectancy of a baby born in a poor country versus one born in the average wealthy nation has shrunk nearly 18 percent.

Alongside the reductions of infectious diseases, the lives of people in poor countries have clearly improved. In 2015, for the first time in history, less than 10 percent of the world's population was living in extreme poverty, defined by the World Bank as living on less than $1.90 per day. Seventy-one percent of the people on the African continent now have access to safe drinking water.[11] The relationship between better health and these broader economic and infrastructure improvements, discussed at greater length in the next chapter, is still much debated. What is certain is that the decline in infectious diseases in lower-income nations is a remarkable achievement, perhaps among the greatest in human history, freeing hundreds of millions of people from the grip of an early death and a life of painful disability.

The present gains against pestilence are different from those in the past. Reductions in infectious disease that took centuries to manifest themselves in countries that are wealthy today took place within a generation or two in still-poor nations. These recent declines in plagues and parasites have also materialized in troubled countries with dysfunctional governments. In Nepal, a poor country only a few years removed from a Maoist insurgency, life expectancy has increased by eleven years since 1990, reaching an average of 70 years in 2015. Many of the other countries that have increased their life expectancy by more than a dozen years would not lead many readers' lists for least troubled nations either: Angola, Equatorial Guinea, Liberia, Maldives, Niger, Rwanda, Timor-Leste, Uganda, and, of course, Ethiopia. Donor-funded, treatment-driven initiatives in Ethiopia and other poor nations have helped achieve remarkable reductions in plagues and parasites in Ethiopia and other poor nations, but have not resulted in the strong public health systems and more responsive governance that generally accompanied infectious disease control elsewhere. The model for these international aid initiatives was first pioneered in military and colonial campaigns against plagues and parasites.

The Colonial and Military Roots of Global Health

For most of human history, plagues, parasites, and pests were a domestic affair. States began negotiating agreements with each other on infectious disease control and sanitation only in the second half of the nineteenth century. This was the same era when governments were concluding international treaties on telegraphy, the postal service, weights and measures, and time zones. The basic purpose of all these treaties was the same: standardization to facilitate trade. Quarantine was the principal means of containing the microbes and plagues that arrived at ports and rail stations, but governments often abused the practice to benefit their own merchants or punish other nations.[12]

The first international agreement on the quarantining of ships and ports was finalized in 1892.[13] In 1902, the International Sanitary Bureau, which later became the Pan American Health Organization, was established to help coordinate infectious disease control.[14] Five years later, the International Office of Public Hygiene was created to oversee quarantine rules and to share statistics from health departments around the world. It had a staff of only a half dozen people and could hardly fulfill its mission.[15] Nations, rich and poor alike, were still largely on their own in confronting the plagues and parasites that ravaged their citizens. As industrialized nations better understood the causes of infectious diseases, they invested more in domestic public health and sanitation and imposed fewer quarantines. Their interest in international health cooperation waned.[16]

International efforts to control infectious disease in poorer nations did not emerge from an enlightened sense of global solidarity in humanity's fight against plagues and parasites. Instead, the roots of global health are in conquest and colonization. More attention has been given to the historical role that the tiny microbes accompanying armies and explorers played in toppling grand empires, but infectious diseases also doomed many expeditions and encumbered colonies. Investing in infectious disease control facilitated conquest, made the tropics habitable for settlers, and improved the productivity of local laborers. It also advanced humanitarian and moral goals of empires and eased tensions between Western colonizers and indigenous peoples.

Today's wealthy governments are still driven by that same mix of self-interest, geostrategic priorities, and humanitarian concern as they seek to address health concerns in poorer nations. Those actions do not always correspond with the biggest sources of death and disability. The colonial and military roots of global health also help explain the way that international aid initiatives traditionally sought to prevent and treat plagues and parasites in developing countries—with scientific interventions deployed in targeted campaigns, rather than through improving local governance or reducing poverty and inequity. A brief history of smallpox and malaria, and the different ways that these diseases were addressed in wealthy and poorer nations, helps tell the story.

The Spotted Plague

Smallpox, one of the greatest killers in human history, is believed to have begun life as a gerbil virus. That virus jumped from those African rodents to people and camels roughly 3,500 years ago and spread along trade routes to the early urban centers of southern Asia and the Nile Delta region.[17] Egyptian mummies dating back to 1155 BCE, including Pharaoh Ramses V, bear telltale pockmark scars that may be the earliest evidence of the disease.[18] In the centuries that followed, smallpox did inestimable damage. In the twentieth century alone, the disease has been estimated to be responsible for as many as 300 million deaths (more than three times the number killed in that century's wars).[19]

The path to smallpox's poxes started with the sufferer inhaling infectious material left from a past victim of the disease. Once inside, the virus entered the lymph nodes, multiplied, and spilled out into the bloodstream. A week or so later, the symptoms began with a headache, fever, pains, and vomiting. Three days after that, the skin erupted in waxy, hard, and painful pustules—spots that spread everywhere, including in the mouth and throat, and pressed together like a "cobblestone street."[20] Bacteria often contaminated those pustules, leading to abscesses and corneal ulcers that could, in turn, lead to blindness. Between 20 and 50 percent of victims perished from the disease, often as a result of septic shock.[21] In regions where smallpox was endemic, it was mostly a threat to children under a year old. Among populations where the disease was unknown, however, all were susceptible.

The risk that smallpox posed to people without prior exposure made it one of history's great diseases of conquest. But that is a view of history told by its victors. Smallpox has also been a major reason for military disaster and disruption of empires, and not just among the Amerindian population. The Huns were repelled from Gaul and Italy by an epidemic of a disease believed to be smallpox, reportedly spread after the beheading of a bishop who was a survivor of the disease. That bishop later became known as Saint Nicaise, the patron saint of smallpox victims.[22] The first major battlefield defeat of the United States occurred after a smallpox epidemic disabled half of the Continental Army at the Siege of Quebec during the early days of the Revolutionary War.[23] Some claim that smallpox is the reason that Canada remains part of the British Commonwealth.[24] A smallpox outbreak saved the British again in 1779, thwarting a naval invasion of England where French and Spanish ships outnumbered their English counterparts by two to one.[25]

Smallpox remained a leading cause of death in Europe into the late eighteenth century; it played a major role in dismantling the secession plans of many royal families. Among those who perished from smallpox were Emperor Joseph I of Austria; King Louis XV of France; Tsar Peter II of Russia; King Luis I of Spain; Queen Ulrika Eleonora of Sweden; and Prince William, the eleven-year-old sole heir of Queen Anne of England, the last of the Stuarts.[26]

In 1796, Edward Jenner developed a vaccine for smallpox derived from a virus that was infecting cows but may have been horsepox.[27] It was the first truly effective medical intervention for preventing an infectious disease. Unsurprisingly, royalty and political leaders in Europe were early to embrace and actively encourage use of the new vaccine. New health laws to promote smallpox vaccination campaigns were adopted, first in northern Italy and Sweden, then in England and Wales, and later in France and Germany. After a smallpox epidemic killed China's emperor, Japan sent a mission to Europe to study vaccine production and adopted compulsory vaccination a few years later.[28] The dowager empress in Russia ordered that the first orphan vaccinated for smallpox be named Vaccinoff and supported for life by the state.[29] In the United States, Thomas Jefferson was an early enthusiast of smallpox vaccination for his young nation, vaccinating himself, his family and neighbors, and the last surviving members of the Mohican tribe, who happened to be visiting.[30]

Immunization programs produced dramatic declines in smallpox deaths in these early adopter nations, but the programs were also victims of their own success.[31] As smallpox rates plummeted, antivaccination campaigns gained ground, especially in immigrant and rural communities wary of state intrusion. Fierce pushback from these groups ensued, particularly in Britain and the United States, and compulsory immunization was scaled back in several nations.[32] The struggle over smallpox immunization forced governments to grapple with the hard balance between ensuring the public good and respecting individual rights.[33] These struggles paved the way for the adoption of other forms of social regulation including compulsory schooling and military service.

Smallpox is also notable as the first disease to have demonstrated the difference that effective infectious disease control could make in war.

The decision of General George Washington, himself a pockmarked survivor of the disease, to inoculate his troops at Valley Forge against smallpox may have saved the colonial war effort against a British army that was less susceptible to the disease.[34] A smallpox outbreak spread by troop movements and refugees from Paris in 1870 during the Franco-Prussian War killed half a million people in Europe, including 20,000 French soldiers, but only 500 of the well-vaccinated and victorious German troops.[35] After the Franco-Prussian War, military and colonial investments in infectious disease control and research increased, especially for mosquito-borne diseases such as malaria.

The Cost of Failing to Outwit a Mosquito

Like smallpox, malaria is an old disease, caused by a parasite that emerged as a major killer of people thousands of years ago, around the advent of agriculture.[36] Malaria is not deadly to the cold-blooded mosquitos that carry it, but the parasite rapidly multiplies in the red blood cells of warm humans and bursts forth, inciting fever and debilitating weakness. When the parasitized red blood cells accumulate and clog the blood vessels of the brain, cerebral malaria ensues, which is fatal if untreated. The fever caused by malaria enables the parasite to move freely in the bloodstream for a day or two, when another mosquito may bite the sufferer and suck up the parasite, starting the cycle anew. The symptoms of malaria are more severe in people without prior exposure to the disease and can be especially deadly for children. Immunity to malaria builds up slowly and is quickly lost without repeated contact. The *Anopheles* mosquitos that carry the malaria parasite do well in any warm weather environment with standing water and thrive in the wells and ditches in villages, military camps, and farms where there are enough people to sustain transmission of the parasite.

The role that malaria has played in history has been as more of a disease of colonies, a hindrance to exploration and settlement, than a help to military conquests. The famed malariologist Paul Russell led the US Army's efforts against the disease in World War II and once wrote of malaria's toll:

> Man ploughs the sea like a leviathan, he soars through the air like an eagle; his voice circles the world in a moment, his eyes pierce the heavens; he moves mountains, he makes the desert to bloom; he has planted his flag at the north pole and the south; yet millions of men each year are destroyed because they fail to outwit a mosquito.[37]

The strain of malaria that is endemic in Africa, *Plasmodium falciparum*, is particularly deadly to outsiders. For centuries, it repelled explorers and would-be conquerors of the continent. In the 1560s and 1570s, Portugal made several attempts to bring missionaries and armies from Europe to Mozambique and expand the empire's African foothold inland, only to see malaria cut down priests and soldiers alike.[38] In 1805, forty-two men accompanied Mungo Park, a Scottish doctor and best-selling author, in his expedition to reach Timbuktu, a city fabled to contain the treasure of Prester John. Forty-one of them died of malaria. Park and one other man survived until an ambush by Tuaregs forced them into a crocodile-infested section of the Niger River. Park's son, Thomas, launched an expedition to find his father and also likely perished of malaria.[39]

Malaria has been hindering armies since the disease kept the Han Dynasty (202 BCE to 221 CE) from expanding into the Yellow River flood plain and the Yangtze Valley.[40] More than a thousand years later, the disease remained a major obstacle to military campaigns. More than a million soldiers suffered malaria during the US Civil War.[41] During World War I, malaria bogged down troops in Macedonia, East Africa, Mesopotamia, and Palestine. In 1918, half of Britain's 40,000 troops pursuing Turkish forces into the Jordan Valley were lost to malaria.[42]

Amid increased colonization and the two world wars of the twentieth century, more research was devoted to malaria and its control, but the fruits of that research emerged only after the disease had already declined precipitously in the prosperous nations of world. In the sixteenth century, malaria was once common enough in England and Northern Europe for the disease's symptoms to earn references in the works of Shakespeare, Dante, and Chaucer. By 1880, however, improved drainage and extensive land reclamation had dramatically reduced the mosquito-friendly marshes that supported the disease. Greater mechanization of agriculture and improvements in rural housing further cut transmission rates.[43]

Progress in the United States also predated the development of effective pesticides for malaria-bearing mosquitos. Starting in 1912, the US Public Health Service, with funding from the Rockefeller Foundation, tested malaria control strategies to determine the most cost-effective approach and generate public support in the American South.[44] Once the benefits of drainage for reducing malaria-spreading mosquitos and improving worker productivity were demonstrated, US public health officials solicited support from local businesses for their expansion. Lawsuits and federal regulations forced the booming US hydropower industry to change the design of dams to clear stagnant waterways and cut mosquito habitats further.[45] By the time effective pesticides were developed and the US Malaria Control in War Areas program (which later became the US Centers for Disease Control and Prevention) began to use them to eliminate mosquitos, malaria rates had already plummeted. The United States went from having more than a million cases of malaria during the Great Depression to effectively eliminating the disease from the country by 1952.[46]

The opportunities for lower-income nations to adopt their own national and local measures to control infectious diseases like malaria and smallpox were limited. Many of these countries were poor, rural, and disrupted by conquest and colonization. The warmer climate in many of these nations meant a higher burden of tropical diseases. Malaria remains endemic today in ninety-one countries and territories, mostly lower-income nations.[47] Smallpox, despite the availability of an effective vaccine, continued to kill hundreds of millions in lower-income nations over the nineteenth and twentieth centuries.[48]

Eradication and the First International Health Campaigns

The first international campaigns to prevent infectious disease in poorer nations were the vaccination expeditions launched by the Spanish and British Empires shortly after Jenner's invention of the smallpox vaccine. The British campaign, launched in 1802, targeted India. The Spanish Royal Philanthropic Vaccine Expedition, which started in 1803, was even more ambitious—a decade-long effort that carried smallpox vaccine from Spain to the Caribbean, to New Spain (Mexico) and Guatemala, to Venezuela, down the Pacific coast of South America and up to its Andean provinces, and to the Philippines and China.[49]

To preserve the smallpox vaccine in warm climates and over long journeys, these early expeditions took advantage of two of its unique properties. First, the smallpox vaccine, unlike most modern vaccines, is a live virus (a hybrid of the smallpox and cowpox or horsepox viruses) that can be delivered through the skin. The vaccine was administered by rubbing it into a series of small cuts made with a knife, called a lancet (in later smallpox immunization campaigns, bifurcated needles were developed for this purpose). After a period of incubation, those cuts erupted into lesions that

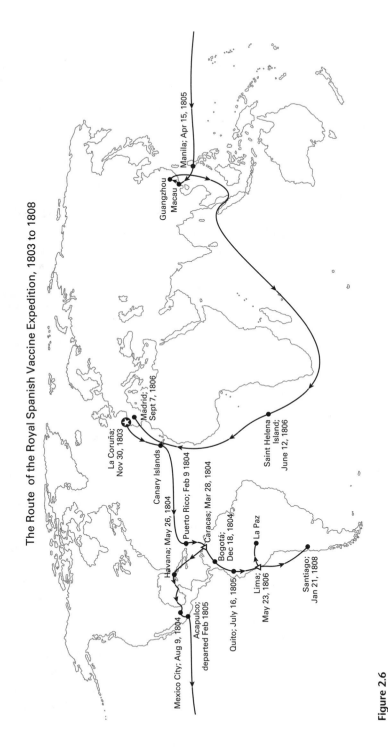

The Route of the Royal Spanish Vaccine Expedition, 1803 to 1808

Figure 2.6

Adapted from Soto-Pérez-de-Celis, "The Royal Philanthropic Expedition of the Vaccine," 2008; Franco-Paredes, Lammoglia, and Santos-Preciado, "The Spanish Royal Philanthropic Expedition," 2005.

oozed fluid brimming with the hybrid virus. That serum could be harvested by squeezing those open lesions and using the fluid that emerged to vaccinate another person. Second, the incubation period before those lesions emerged was long, nine or ten days, which meant that only a few dozen passengers on these expeditions, instead of hundreds, could be used to sustain and relay the vaccine arm-to-arm around the world.

The passengers chosen for this purpose were orphans, some as young as five years old. A relay of children brought the smallpox vaccine arm-to-arm from Baghdad to Bombay to launch the British immunization campaign in India. Twenty-one Spanish orphans were used to transport the vaccine on the two-month journey from Spain to the Caribbean in 1804. The director of the orphanage, and the only woman aboard, also brought her son so that he might contribute to the mission.[50] The process of harvesting the vaccine could lead to infections and fatal complications, and the British Sanitary Commissioner for Bengal reported that the "agony caused to the child was often intense."[51] Four of the children who participated in the Spanish voyages died.[52] In later vaccination campaigns, calves were used to transport and harvest the vaccine before heat-stable and freeze-dried versions were invented decades later.[53]

These early vaccination campaigns had multiple purposes. The British and Spanish governments saw these missions as opportunities to generate goodwill and demonstrate the benefits of colonization at a time when there were few other cures or prophylactics for infectious disease. A healthier workforce increased the productivity of colonies, which depended on agriculture, textile production, and other labor-intensive activities.[54] The safety of colonial officials also depended on the vaccination of those around them.[55] But humanitarian interests were also at work.[56] Charles IV (the Bourbon King of Spain) was committed to spreading the benefits of vaccination to the Spanish empire after his brother died of smallpox and his daughter was infected with the virus.[57] Overall, the Spanish and British vaccine expeditions are estimated to have vaccinated as many as half a million people.[58]

International initiatives against malaria in lower-income nations began with colonial and army physicians working to address surges in the disease that colonization itself had helped cause. A growing demand for raw materials spurred the industrializing powers of Europe and the United States to shift their colonies to mining and plantation-style farms, and to build canals to transport the produced commodities. These changes transformed the physical landscape and concentrated large numbers of local laborers in settings conducive to the spread of malaria.[59] As colonial governments expanded and civilian and military staffs grew, garrison hospitals and medical centers were established. These facilities mostly served Europeans, but sometimes had special wards for "natives."[60] The army and colonial doctors assigned to those sites later emerged as the first practitioners of tropical medicine, a new discipline focused on infectious and parasitic diseases.[61]

In 1880, Charles Laveran, a French physician working in a military hospital in Constantine, Algeria, discovered that a parasite caused malaria, rather than, as previously thought, the foul water and bad air that gave the disease its name (*mal aria*). Sir Ronald Ross, a British army surgeon working in Calcutta (now Kolkata), India, discovered that mosquitos carried the parasite in their salivary glands and spread the disease through bites. Colonial and military health officials founded research institutions like the Liverpool and London Schools of Tropical Medicine, which developed the strategies to control malaria and trained generations of infectious disease specialists.[62]

One adopter of these strategies was William Crawford Gorgas, an Alabama-born army surgeon. He used the discoveries of Ronald Ross on malaria, and related research by Walter Reed about yellow fever, to conduct the first practical demonstrations of disease eradication via antimosquito campaigns. The ravages of malaria and yellow fever had thwarted French efforts to build a canal in Panama connecting the Pacific and Atlantic oceans. As the chief sanitary officer of the US-led Panama Canal Commission between 1904 and 1913, Gorgas drained one hundred square miles of territory, applied millions of gallons of oil and kerosene to kill breeding sites, and paid children to hand-kill adult mosquitos. The campaign worked, cutting malaria cases by 80 percent, eliminating yellow fever, and allowing the successful construction of the canal.[63] When Gorgas began his work, the death rate in the Canal Zone was three times higher than the continental United States; by the time he finished in 1915, the death rate in the Canal Zone had fallen to half that in the United States.[64] Gorgas, together with former colonial health officers and veterans of the US Army Medical Corps, took this approach of military-style, single disease campaigns with them to the Rockefeller Foundation and the first international health institutions.[65]

The League of Nations was founded in the aftermath of World War I to prevent future wars through collective security, disarmament, and international

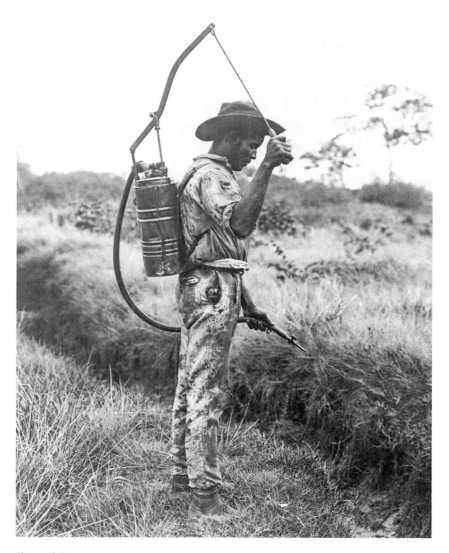

Figure 2.7
A man spraying oil on mosquito breeding grounds in Panama. Reprinted with
permission from the Library of Congress.

arbitration of disputes. As part of that mission, the League established a health section that became known as the League of Nations Health Organization. That organization established a malaria commission in 1924 to assess and advance antimalarial strategies to address war-related surges of the disease in southern Europe, an effort that eventually expanded to Latin America and the Caribbean, and parts of Asia.[66]

World War II spurred a furious expansion of those antimalarial strategies. Germany's invasion of the Netherlands and the Japanese conquest of Java blocked the Allied powers' access to quinine, the only effective antimalarial drug at the time, which was produced on Dutch-owned plantations in Indonesia.[67] As the war pushed into the malarial zones of the Pacific and Mediterranean, the toll of disease mounted. At one point, in the early stages of the war, General Douglas MacArthur estimated that two-thirds of his troops in the South Pacific were ill with malaria.[68] Whole divisions fell sick to the disease in the Battle of Bataan, helping the Japanese defeat US and Philippine forces. The American Forces Radio in the South Pacific broadcast so many messages about avoiding malaria that US troops dubbed it the "Mosquito Network."[69] In 1943, the US Army even drafted Dr. Seuss, writing under his real name Theodor Geisel, to pen a mildly racy cartoon pamphlet about avoiding the bites of *Anopheles* mosquitos. It begins with a keyhole view of a seductively posed mosquito and the line "Ann really gets around." Despite those efforts, five hundred thousand US GIs are estimated to have contracted malaria during World War II.[70]

The US antimalarial research program at Johns Hopkins University tested thousands of compounds before developing chloroquine, the first new treatment of the disease since Jesuit missionaries documented the medicinal properties of cinchona tree bark (quinine) in the 1630s.[71] The insecticide DDT was first tested as a means of controlling lice-borne typhus during the Allied liberation of Naples in October 1943 and used against malaria in the US Marines' assault on Peleliu and Saipan.[72] The success of those efforts led the United States to approve DDT for civilian use after the war.[73] The insecticide was so effective that the last remaining malaria cases were eradicated from the United States in 1952 and, a few years later, from most of Europe.[74] Its inventor, Paul Müller, won a Nobel Prize for his work on DDT in 1948.

The medical advances of World War II, combined with the development of antibiotics and vaccines beyond smallpox, facilitated rapid responses to

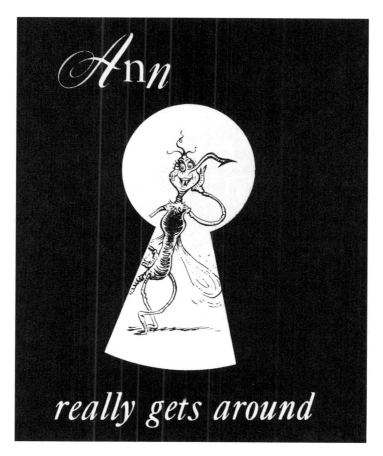

Figure 2.8
Theodor S. Geisel, *This Is Ann: She's Dying to Meet You*. Pamphlet,
Washington, DC: United States Government Printing Office, 1943.

disease threats and made unnecessary the slow, broad-based path that developed nations had pursued to better health.[75] The horrors of World War II also inspired commitment in global leaders to build new forms of international cooperation to promote economic development and confront the humanitarian crisis left after the conflict. The World Health Organization (WHO) was established as part of the United Nations in 1946 and given a broad mandate to promote health. But it was not given the resources to match. Cold War tensions between the United States and the Soviet Union pushed the WHO to focus on rapid, high-impact infectious disease control programs, with the goal of helping to win the hearts and minds of developing nations, many of them beginning to throw off their colonial chains.[76]

US support and the success of the DDT-led campaigns helped push the WHO to launch a global malaria eradication program in 1955, the first effort to eradicate an infectious disease from the face of the earth. Three years later, with the support of the Soviet Union, the WHO began a campaign to eradicate smallpox as well.

The goal of the WHO's malaria campaign was to interrupt transmission of the disease by spraying DDT to kill the mosquitos that spread the disease and to identify and treat all those with the disease to prevent returning mosquitos from becoming reinfected. Within a decade, the campaign eliminated malaria from twenty-six countries—more than half of the nations participating in the campaign. In the other countries, malaria rates were driven down dramatically.[77] But some of that progress was later reversed as mosquitos became resistant to DDT and use of the pesticide was stopped worldwide over environmental concerns (largely from the overuse of the insecticide in wealthy countries' agriculture). By 1969, the WHO was forced to admit that the malaria campaign would never achieve its global goal of eradicating the disease, a major blow to the institution and its prestige. Still, by the time it was canceled, the malaria eradication program had protected an estimated 1.1 billion people from the disease at a cost of $1.4 billion over ten years, or roughly $10 billion in today's terms.[78]

The smallpox eradication program accomplished even more for less. Smallpox had several advantages over malaria as a target for eradication. While smallpox still killed an estimated two million people per year in the late 1950s, it was endemic only in Brazil, India, Pakistan, Afghanistan, Nepal, Indonesia, and most of sub-Saharan Africa.[79] The distinct pocking that the disease caused and the manner in which it spread (person to person, rather than via mosquitos) made smallpox easier to identify, track, and ultimately wipe out. Nevertheless, the smallpox campaign languished for years at the WHO with little support. A major turning point came in 1965 when President Lyndon Johnson, who needed an initiative to announce to mark the United Nations' "International Cooperation Year," threw the United States' support behind an intensified antismallpox campaign, which was launched two years later.[80]

Ten years of heroic work and more than 370 million vaccine doses later, the eradication campaign brought the number of smallpox cases to zero.

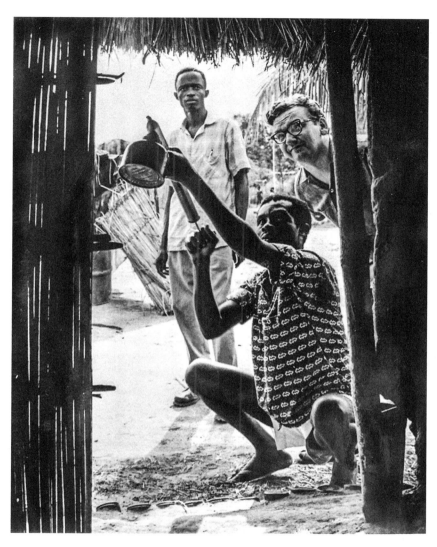

Figure 2.9
Pasquale Caprari, WHO scientist, supervises malaria-campaign workers spraying a hut with DDT in Ghana in 1950. Photo: WHO/UN, Courtesy of WHO.

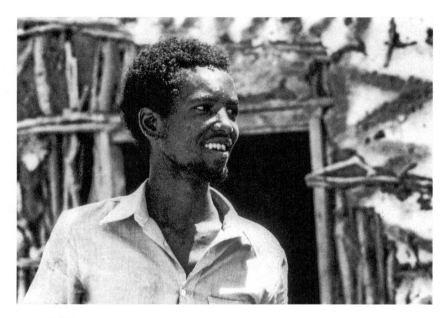

Figure 2.10
Ali Maow Maalin, who contracted the world's last recorded case of endemic
smallpox, pictured here in 1979. Photo: WHO/John F. Wickett, Courtesy of WHO.

Ethiopia was the last country in the world where smallpox was endemic.
The last case of smallpox was found on October 26, 1977, across Ethiopia's
border with Somalia, in a hospital cook named Ali Maow Maalin working
in the town of Merka.[81] The cost of the intensified smallpox eradication
campaign was $313 million.[82] In 1980, the World Health Assembly declared
"the world and all its peoples have won freedom from smallpox, which
was a most devastating disease sweeping in epidemic form through many
countries since earliest times, leaving death, blindness, and disfigurement
in its wake and which only a decade ago was rampant in Africa, Asia and
South America."[83]

The legacy of the smallpox campaign extends beyond that disease.
Many of the men and women who directed that effort—D. A. Henderson, Bill Foege, David Heymann, and others—later became leaders in the
new field of global health. The smallpox campaign is also remembered for
demonstrating the viability of a new model for improving health in poor
nations that was disease specific, coordinated by international agencies and

infectious disease specialists, and implemented by local staff and volunteers. That approach is now known as a "vertical" program because it is directed internationally (from above) and targets just one disease, often with a single intervention such as a vaccine.[84]

Adoption of this approach to improving global health was not inevitable. The first director of the International Health Division of the Rockefeller Foundation, Wickliffe Rose, argued that the purpose of the foundation should not be to eradicate a particular disease, but to demonstrate the benefits of professionally run public health programs to inspire local agencies and policymakers to take up that cause permanently.[85] He was overruled and ultimately pushed out, with Frederick Gates, Rockefeller's philanthropy advisor, arguing that Rose's mission was one that "a thousand years will not accomplish."[86]

Day-to-day innovations and adaptations of local officials in fact played a significant role in the success of the smallpox eradication campaign in countries like India.[87] Some WHO staff advocated that the smallpox eradication campaign should work more through local health centers to build up the capability of basic health services. But that strategy, whatever its long-term benefits may have been, cost more and resulted in lower vaccination rates.[88] The vertical model, which first evolved from colonial and military efforts to control threatening tropical diseases, continues to prove remarkably effective in reducing the rates of targeted infectious diseases. That progress has not, however, been accompanied by the broader gains in responsive governance that occurred with infectious disease control in the past.

The Path to Better Health in Poorer Nations

Not all the progress against infectious diseases in lower-income nations after World War II relied on international aid campaigns or medical inventions. China, Costa Rica, and Sri Lanka, among others, found cheap and ingenious ways of preventing infectious disease. Many but not all of these first-mover governments were socialist and, at the time, based their legitimacy on their ability to improve health, education, and literacy for the masses. These nations benefited from the technical support of the WHO, but their biggest health gains were achieved through homegrown, low-cost strategies. These methods included training peasants from the community to serve as health extension workers, dig pit latrines, assist with births, and extract the parasite-carrying snails that lived in the trenches around villages.[89] Between 1946 and 1953, life expectancy in Sri Lanka rose twelve years.[90] Life expectancy in Jamaica and Malaysia increased by a year annually for more than a decade.[91] These health gains occurred well before the economic growth that China and these countries would later achieve.[92]

But most of the reduction in plagues and parasites that occurred in developing nations after World War II was dependent on antibiotics, vaccines, and, to a lesser extent, aid. This was in part a matter of timing. Effective medicines were available when these countries began their health transitions, and so the governments and health workers of these nations put those medicines to good use.[93] The demographer Samuel Preston estimates that vaccines and antibiotics drove half of the declines in death rates in developing countries through the late 1970s.[94] Foreign aid played a small but important role in these early successes, developing new low-cost health measures, training medical personnel, and expanding access to effective medicines. Income was more important than before; emerging countries with greater wealth could afford to spend more on vaccines, antibiotics, and improvements in obstetrics. Child mortality fell by 75 percent or more in Latin America, East Asia, and the Middle East by 2000, a spectacular rate of decline that far exceeds what had occurred in wealthy nations. The health gains extended even to countries with nascent public health systems, poor living conditions, and high rates of malnutrition.[95]

But many developing countries, especially the poorest and most conflict-ridden, lagged behind. In 1990, there were nearly two dozen countries where as many as 175 children out of 1,000 died before the age of five and infectious diseases caused the majority of death and disability.[96] Dramatic improvements in the health of these poorest nations would come only after the international response to HIV/AIDS, an epidemic that, at one time, had threatened to wipe out all the health gains that preceded it.

HIV/AIDS transformed global health, elevating infectious diseases as a foreign policy priority and helping to mobilize billions of dollars to research, develop, and distribute new medicines to meet the needs of the world's most impoverished people. The HIV epidemic, which began in the 1980s, has been responsible for 35 million deaths worldwide (as of the end of 2016).[97] More than two-thirds of HIV cases and three-quarters of HIV deaths took place on the African continent.[98] At its height, the epidemic reduced life expectancy by up to fifteen years in several sub-Saharan African countries. A quarter of all adults in Botswana, Swaziland, and Lesotho contracted the disease. It wasn't until 1998 that an international crisis emerged as it became publicized that many people in sub-Saharan Africa and other lower-income nations were dying without access to the life-saving treatments that had changed the course of the HIV/AIDS epidemic in wealthy nations.

Two developments sparked that international controversy. First, global trade talks established the World Trade Organization (WTO) and led to commitments that member countries must adopt minimum standards of intellectual property protection including patents on medicines. Second, life-saving antiretroviral medicines were developed for HIV/AIDS in response to the outbreak of the disease in the United States and Europe.

Pharmaceutical companies, concerned about undercutting their developed country markets, adopted internationally consistent prices for these drugs. In 1998, antiretroviral drugs cost more in South Africa, on a per capita GDP-adjusted basis, than in Sweden or the United States.[99] Protests spread, disrupting international HIV/AIDS conferences and WTO meetings in Seattle in 1999.[100] Trade disputes and court battles ensued over compulsory licenses, a tool that allows governments to circumvent a patent without the consent of its owner. Popular support for the pharmaceutical industry and international trade plummeted.

Amid the crisis, international investment in improving the health of developing countries began to rise. Aid to address infectious diseases in poor countries rose more than 10 percent annually over the next decade, expanding from $10.8 billion to $28.2 billion.[101] Funding for research into new treatments for HIV/AIDS, malaria, tuberculosis, and other infectious diseases rose thirty-fold over that time, to more than $3 billion.[102] The US government, the Bill and Melinda Gates Foundation, and other donors established new programs to provide drugs and vaccines to the world's poorest. These included the Global Alliance for Vaccines and Immunization (Gavi) in 2000; the Global Fund to Fight AIDS, Tuberculosis, and Malaria (Global Fund) in 2002; and the US President's Emergency Plan for AIDS Relief (PEPFAR) in 2003. Drug companies and universities donated or voluntarily licensed their patents on medicines to treat infectious diseases for which there was little demand in wealthy markets. Competition and voluntary price cuts reduced the price of antiretroviral treatment in poor countries from $12,000 per year in 1996 to $200 per year in 2004.[103] More than ten million people living with HIV/AIDS in sub-Saharan Africa are on those lifesaving medicines today, up from just one hundred thousand in 2003.[104]

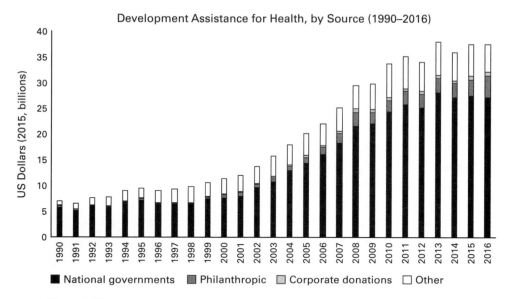

Figure 2.11

Data source: Institute for Health Metrics and Evaluation, *Financing for Global Health* (2016).

Together, these efforts have delivered treatments, insecticide-treated mosquito nets, and immunization to millions, dramatically reducing the burden of plagues and parasites and saving many lives. Infectious diseases are no longer the leading causes of years of life lost to death and disability globally. Since 2005, rates of the infectious diseases targeted by global health initiatives, like HIV, malaria, measles, and Guinea worm, have been the ones to decline the fastest.

Amid this welcome progress, however, are worrisome signs for the future of international health initiatives. An idiosyncratic mix of motivations fueled the recent surge in investments to fight infectious diseases. As in the era of conquest and colony, some of these motivations were humanitarian and some were geostrategic. In deciding to launch the PEPFAR program, President George W. Bush reportedly asked how the United States would be judged if it did not act to address a preventable and treatable epidemic of such magnitude.[105] Increasing US global health spending also promoted positive views of the country on the African continent, at a time when the United States had launched an unpopular war in Iraq.[106] Massive protests over pricey HIV/AIDS medicines also brought global attention to a long-standing problem—international systems for medical research and development were not responding to the health needs of developing countries—and spurred the drug industry and its supporters to do more to defuse the issue.[107]

This confluence of motivations has proven difficult to replicate in response to other global health challenges. As a result, while the burden of many infectious diseases has changed in poorer nations, the distribution of international aid targeting these diseases has not. For example, 30 percent of development assistance for health is still focused on HIV/AIDS, which is now responsible for 5 percent of the death and disability in lower-income nations.[108]

International AIDS programs have invested in partnerships, clinics, and local health personnel to deliver antiretroviral drugs and related services in lower-income nations, but they largely remain vertical, disease-specific programs. Even global health programs with wider objectives, such as improved maternal, newborn, and child health, have mostly followed the same vertical approach as the old eradication programs rather than investing in strengthening countries' health systems.[109]

Health spending has increased in lower-income nations, but relative to wealthy countries, it remains low.[110] All forty-eight governments in sub-Saharan Africa together spent less on health in 2014 ($67 billion) than the government of Australia ($68 billion).[111] Health spending that same year by all low- and middle-income country governments, representing 5.9 billion people, was roughly the same spent by the governments of the United States and Canada, with a combined population of 360 million.[112] In fact, research by economists Joe Dieleman and Michael Hanlon suggests that the governments of poor countries are shifting their resources away from the health areas targeted by aid donors.[113]

In many countries in Africa, Latin America, and Asia, rural patients must still travel long distances to get treatment even for common conditions. The government-run hospitals offer affordable or free care but are often overcrowded and understaffed. Basic medical equipment, such as rehydration fluids, disposable syringes, gauze, and the like, may be unavailable. More expensive machinery like X-ray machines and MRI scanners are often inadequately maintained.[114] In many countries, medicines are still purchased out of pocket and are often beyond the means of poor households.[115] Inadequate oversight of antibiotic use and overcrowding in hospitals in Bangladesh, Pakistan, and other lower-income nations is spurring resistance to medicines that helped make possible the recent miraculous gains against infectious diseases.[116] Private investment is increasing in hospitals in India, Nigeria, Ethiopia, and a few lower-income nations, but that investment to date mostly benefits the small wealthy and middle classes.[117]

Given strained public health systems, limited personal wealth, and modest government health spending, many lower-income countries are vulnerable to health challenges that have historically not attracted much donor funding.

Death and Demography

A sunny equatorial climate and the perceived abundance of available land began drawing English settlers to start farms in Kenya, Uganda, and Tanzania in the 1920s. Scores of British doctors followed, working in government service or in missionary hospitals. In their free time, these British doctors did what British doctors often do: they started medical journals. The early pages of the *Kenya Medical Journal* and other publications were consumed with a great medical mystery: whether Africans were naturally predisposed to lifelong low blood pressure. A case of hypertension had never been recorded in the region and would not be seen until the early 1940s. Obesity was rare enough that Sir Julian Huxley, a British biologist, recorded with amazement that the only overweight person he saw in four months in East Africa was a woman who worked in the Nairobi brewery, causing him to entertain the possibility that beer might be fattening.[118]

Today, it is far easier to find cases of heart disease and obesity in sub-Saharan Africa. In fact, heart disease, cancers, diabetes, and other noncommunicable diseases are increasing rapidly in most developing countries.[119] In 1990, these noncommunicable diseases caused about a quarter of the death and disability in poor nations. By 2040, that number is expected to jump to as high as 80 percent in some of these countries. At that point, the burden of heart disease and other noncommunicable diseases in Ethiopia, Bangladesh, and Myanmar will be roughly the same as it will be in rich nations such as the United States and the United Kingdom. The difference is that shift from infectious diseases to noncommunicable diseases took roughly three to four times as long in those wealthy countries.[120]

Fewer people dying as children and adolescents from plagues and parasites helps explain why more people in lower-income countries are getting

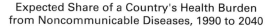

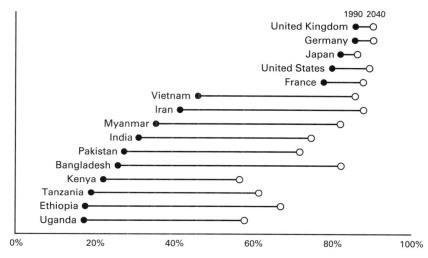

Expected Share of a Country's Health Burden
from Noncommunicable Diseases, 1990 to 2040

Figure 2.12
Source: Bollyky et al., *Health Affairs* (2017).

these noncommunicable diseases. People must ultimately die of something and, if it is not infectious diseases, it is more likely that death will come as a result of noncommunicable disease than via an accident, injury, or violence.

Reductions in plagues and parasites, however, do not explain why so many people in lower-income countries are developing these chronic ailments at much younger ages and with much worse outcomes than in wealthier nations. Premature deaths from hypertensive heart disease (in people age 59 or younger) have increased by nearly 50 percent in sub-Saharan Africa since 1990.[121] The increase of premature heart disease and other chronic illnesses in developing countries is not merely the by-product of rising incomes, or adoption of unhealthy Western lifestyles. Low-income countries are, by past standards, still quite poor. When these nations, most in sub-Saharan Africa, finally achieved an average life expectancy of 60 in 2011, their median GDP per capita ($1,072) was a quarter of the wealth that the residents of high-income countries possessed when they reached that same average life-expectancy in 1947 ($4,334).[122] Unhealthy habits, such as physical inactivity and consumption of fatty foods, are increasing in poor countries, but are still much rarer than in middle-income and rich nations.

The rapid increase of noncommunicable diseases in poorer countries is the by-product of the way that infectious diseases have declined in those countries. In earlier transitions, as childhood health improved, so did adult health, though at a more modest pace. Between the late eighteenth century and the start of World War I, for example, the risk of death among people over 30 years old in France decreased by roughly 25 percent.[123] Adult health also advanced in the wave of developing countries that reduced infectious diseases after World War II. In contrast, there has been relatively minimal progress in the health of adults, ages 15 to 50, in those lower-income nations that have experienced more recent health transitions, other than the donor-supported reductions in deaths due to HIV/AIDS.

In fact, the gap in adult life expectancies between poor and wealthy countries has grown. A 15-year-old today in an average low-income country has the same life expectancy as a 15-year-old in that same country in 1990. Meanwhile, a teenager of the same age in a high-income country has a life expectancy of 80 years, five years longer than a similarly placed individual in 1990. That growing global disparity in adult health holds true even if one controls for HIV/AIDS.

The lack of progress in adult health does not bode well for lower-income countries and their aging populations. Figure 2.13 summarizes the death and disability caused by four key diseases since 1990 by country income group. For working-age adults, the likelihood of surviving diseases like stroke

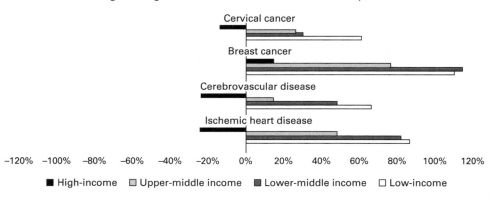

Figure 2.13
Data source: Institute for Health Metrics and Evaluation, GBD 2015.

(cerebrovascular disease) or cervical cancer depends on the wealth of the country where a person lives.[124] The risk of early death from heart disease, diabetes, and many other noncommunicable illnesses, once known as diseases of affluence, now has a stronger statistical link to the poverty of the country than do HIV/AIDS, dengue fever, and many other infectious diseases.[125]

Unfortunately, this problem will only get worse with the shifting demographics of many developing countries. The population growth in many of these nations is much faster than the rates in Europe, the United States, and other wealthy nations when infectious diseases began to decline. In those earlier transitions, population growth rarely exceeded 1 percent per year. This meant that the population of a typical European nation grew three to five times between 1750 and 1950. In the recent transitions in developing countries, population growth rates have often exceeded 2.5 or even 3 percent per year, doubling population in just a decade or two. The number of working-age adults (15 to 64) in many of these poorer countries increased by 15 percent or more every five years.[126]

This means that, even if mortality rates of heart disease (deaths per 1,000 people) do not get worse in many poorer nations, the number of people who survive into adulthood and are more likely to get heart disease and other noncommunicable diseases will still grow spectacularly fast.[127] For example, the median age in Bangladesh, a low-income country, increased from 18 to 26 years between 1990 and 2015. Over the same time, its population increased by more than fifty percent. As a result, there are now more than 38 million additional adults between the ages of 25 and 64 in Bangladesh than there were just twenty-five years ago.[128] As a result, the share of the health burden in Bangladesh due to noncommunicable diseases such as heart disease grew from 26 percent in 1990 to 61 percent in 2015. In Ethiopia, similar demographic changes have driven the noncommunicable disease burden to more than double in twenty-five years; these diseases are now expected to represent the majority of that country's health needs in 2030. Similarly dramatic shifts are happening in other poor countries like Kenya, Myanmar, Nicaragua, and Tanzania. The transition from infectious diseases to noncommunicable ailments such as heart disease in these and other lower-income countries is occurring, and is expected to continue to occur, at a staggeringly fast rate, more rapidly than the world has ever seen before.[129]

Noncommunicable diseases are largely chronic and require more health-care infrastructure and trained health workers than most infectious diseases, and are more costly to treat.[130] A 2013 study in Tanzania estimated that chronic diseases, like cancer and heart disease, were responsible for a quarter of the country's health burden but nearly half of all its hospital admissions and days spent in the hospital.[131] Other studies have shown that inpatient surgical procedures are used more than twice as often for noncommunicable diseases than for infectious diseases.[132] Another study found that the developing countries that are experiencing the fastest transition from infectious to noncommunicable diseases are also the same nations that are least prepared for it.[133] This is particularly true of most sub-Saharan African nations.

To date, neither domestic health spending nor aid budgets are filling this gap. The average government of a low-income country, such as Ethiopia, spends $23 per person annually on health. The typical government of a lower middle-income nation—India, Vietnam, or Nigeria—spends a bit more: $133 per person. In comparison, the United States spends $3,860 per person and the United Kingdom devotes $2,695 per person on health. Most aid donors are not interested in tackling chronic ailments like diabetes and heart disease.[134] In 2011, the United Nations General Assembly held a high-level meeting to mobilize action to address the rising rates of noncommunicable diseases. Dozens of heads of states and thousands of NGOs came. Five years later, annual aid for noncommunicable diseases remains largely unchanged, at $475 million, which is a little over 1 percent of the aid spent each year on health worldwide.[135]

The situation seems poised to worsen as consumption of tobacco products, alcohol, and processed food and beverages increases in poorer nations. Supermarkets and multinational food companies have penetrated every region of the world, even rural areas.[136] Access to fresh fruits and vegetables has declined, especially in East and Southeast Asia and sub-Saharan Africa.[137] Between 1970 and 2000, cigarette consumption tripled in developing countries.[138]

Many developing countries do not yet have the basic consumer protections and public health regulations to cope with these changes.[139] Many of these lower-income nations are relatively small consumer markets, and their governments have limited leverage to demand changes in the labeling and ingredients of food, alcohol, and tobacco products produced for global consumption. Large multinational corporations often have more resources than the governments that oversee them. The market capitalization of

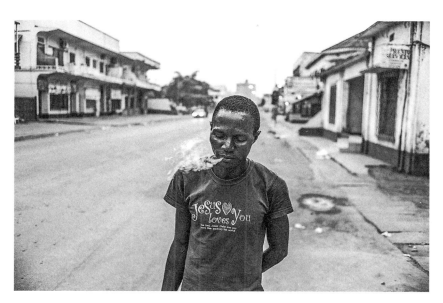

Figure 2.14
Man smoking a cigarette in Bangui, Central African Republic, on February 14, 2014.
Photo: Fred Dufour/AFP/Getty Images.

Philip Morris International at $187 billion (as of July 2017) is larger in nominal terms than the economies of most of the 180 countries where that company sells Marlboro and its other brands of cigarettes.

Tobacco companies, in particular, have been especially aggressive in pursuing teens and women in poor nations, using billboards, cartoons, music sponsorships, and other marketing methods long banned in developed countries.[140] When Uruguay, Togo, and Namibia proposed restrictions on cigarette advertising and labeling, multinational tobacco companies sued under trade and investment agreements to block or delay implementation.[141] These tactics have helped raise tobacco sales across Asia, Eastern Europe, Latin America, and, more recently, Africa.

With little access to preventive care and more exposure to these health risks, working-age people in sub-Saharan Africa and other lower-income nations are more likely to develop cancers, heart diseases, and other noncommunicable diseases than those in wealthy nations. Without access to chronic care and limited household resources to pay for medical treatment out of pocket, these people are also more likely to become disabled or die young.

Share of Death and Disability from Noncommunicable Disease Arising in People under 60

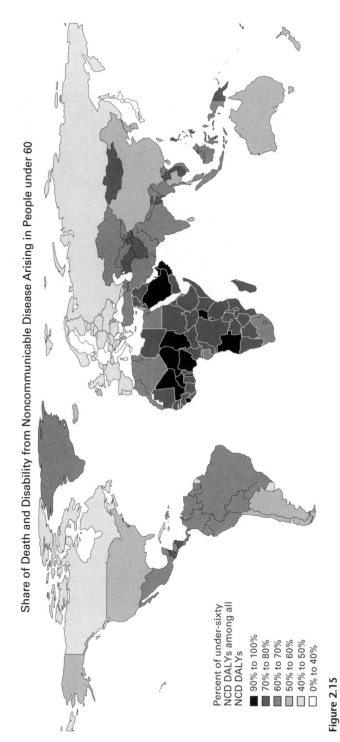

Percent of under-sixty
NCD DALYs among all
NCD DALYs

- ■ 90% to 100%
- 70% to 80%
- 60% to 70%
- 50% to 60%
- 40% to 50%
- □ 0% to 40%

Figure 2.15

Data source: Institute for Health Metrics and Evaluation, GBD 2015.

In sum, the biggest global health crisis in low- and middle-income countries is not the one you might think. It is not the exotic parasites, bacterial blights, and obscure tropical viruses that have long been the focus of international health initiatives and occupied media attention. In 2015 alone, the everyday diseases—cancers, heart diseases, diabetes, and other noncommunicable diseases—killed eight million people before their sixtieth birthdays in low- and middle-income countries. The World Economic Forum projects that noncommunicable diseases will inflict $21.3 trillion in losses in developing countries between 2011 and 2030—a cost that is almost equal to the total aggregate economic output ($26 trillion in constant 2010 US dollars) of these countries in 2015.

The Legacy of Ebola

There are other threats to global health that have exposed the limits of the way the world has gotten better. In December 2013, Emile Ouamouno, a two-year-old boy from Meliandou, Guinea, became ill. He had fever, vomiting, and black stools. His mother cared for the boy, but he died four days later and was buried in his village. A few days later, his mother became sick with the same symptoms and died, as did Emile's sister two weeks later. His grandmother, also sick and understandably alarmed, sought help in Guéckédou, a nearby city with trade links to neighboring Liberia and Sierra Leone. The nurse who treated her had no medical supplies and could do nothing for her. Emile's grandmother returned to Meliandou and died. The first reports of an outbreak surfaced in late January but did not prevent the grandmother's nurse, who also became ill, from traveling to neighboring Macenta for medical care. The nurse died there and the physician who treated him also became ill. Médecins Sans Frontières (Doctors Without Borders) reached Guéckédou to investigate and sent samples for analysis to a laboratory in Lyon, France, which, on March 20, confirmed the deaths were caused by the Ebola virus. Later that same day, the US Centers for Disease Control and Prevention (CDC) announced an outbreak was underway in Guinea, Liberia, and Sierra Leone.[142]

The international response to the outbreak was slow. Part of the reason was that, before the 2013 outbreak, Ebola had killed fewer than 2,000 people over twenty-eight past outbreaks—all in Central Africa.[143] Ebola, which was first identified in 1976, is a terrifying disease, but it does not spread easily. A person with measles, which is an airborne disease, infects eighteen other people on average; a person with Ebola, which is passed through contact with bodily fluids, infects fewer than two other people on average.[144] Ebola also kills quickly in resource-poor countries, which leaves the unfortunate victim with less opportunity to spread it.

But by the time the WHO declared the end of the "public health emergency of international concern" for Ebola on March 29, 2016, the disease had killed 11,323 people and caused 28,646 confirmed cases of infection.[145] The outbreak nearly spread to Nigeria after a foreign diplomat arrived ill at Lagos airport and was taken to a private hospital, where he was correctly diagnosed as having Ebola. A US CDC Emergency Operations Center working together with the Nigerian government was able to trace the nine health workers who came in contact with that official.[146] Had the Ebola virus spread to the sprawling, crowded slums of Lagos, an even greater tragedy might have unfolded.

The eight cases of Ebola that did spread beyond West Africa, however, were enough to cause an international panic. Images of international health workers in cumbersome protective gear amid terrified children and grief-stricken relatives of Ebola victims in West Africa dominated nightly news broadcasts. More than a third of the flights from cities in Europe were canceled and purchases of Ebola survival kits soared in the US Midwest.[147] The outbreak was a topic of debate in US congressional elections. The most recent World Bank estimates reveal that Sierra Leone, Liberia, and Guinea lost $1.6 billion in economic output in 2015 alone, more than 12 percent of their combined GDP.[148]

The difference between the recent Ebola outbreak and its predecessors? Many of the same factors that are increasing the rates of noncommunicable diseases in poorer nations. With greater trade and travel to and within the region, emerging infectious diseases like Ebola are less likely to burn out in rural villages and more likely to reach the still-poor crowded cities with limited health systems that are ideal incubators for outbreaks. As with noncommunicable diseases, long-standing efforts to mobilize more donor support for pandemic preparedness went nowhere, leaving poor nations without the resources to build their capability to monitor and contain disease outbreaks.[149]

Starting in the mid-1990s, WHO and its member governments began revamping the global framework for responding to dangerous infectious disease events, known as the International Health Regulations. That revision granted WHO new powers, including the ability to rely on data from

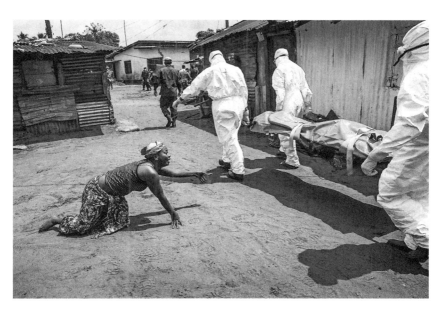

Figure 2.16
A woman crawls toward Ebola burial team members taking the body of her sister away on October 10, 2014, in Monrovia, Liberia. Photo: John Moore/Getty Images.

non-state actors and to issue scientifically grounded advice on responding to outbreaks. The revised International Health Regulations also required countries to monitor, control, and report infectious disease outbreaks. But the resources to support these functions and responsibilities have not been forthcoming.

The portion of the WHO's budget that is funded by dues from 194 member countries is less than the budget of the New York City Department of Health. The other voluntary contributions that WHO receives are earmarked and historically have not prioritized epidemic and pandemic preparedness in poor countries. In 2013, less than 0.5 percent of international health aid was devoted to building global response to infectious disease outbreaks.[150] This has meant that pandemic preparedness has remained largely as it was in the nineteenth century—a domestic affair.

Many lower-income countries are unprepared to assume that burden or adapt to the other changes that have come with declining infectious disease rates. A third of the WHO member nations had implemented their core obligations under the International Health Regulations by 2014.[151] The West African nations most affected by Ebola were not among them.

Prior to the outbreak, Guinea, Liberia, and Sierra Leone had all made commendable progress in reducing the burden of infectious disease in their countries and improving child survival, especially considering the protracted periods of war and instability in the region in the 1990s. Child mortality rates were still high, but had declined at least 33 percent in all three countries since 2002.[152] Sierra Leone boosted its coverage of basic childhood immunizations from 53 percent in 2002 to 93 percent in 2012. Measles immunization rates, an indicator often cited as a basic measure of health performance, rose to 83 percent in Sierra Leone, 74 percent in Liberia, and 62 percent in Guinea. Average life expectancy had improved to 58 years in Guinea and 61 years in Liberia.[153] In the decade before the Ebola outbreak, Guinea, Liberia, and Sierra Leone received nearly $1 billion from the President's Emergency Plan for AIDS Relief, the President's Malaria Initiative, the World Bank, and the Global Fund to Fight AIDS, Tuberculosis, and Malaria.

These donor investments saved many lives, but unfortunately did little to build capable health systems in these countries to respond to other health threats and needs. Before the Ebola outbreak, the governments of Guinea, Liberia, and Sierra Leone still spent little on health: $9, $20, and $16 per person each year, respectively. Many health services were provided by local staff of donor- and faith-based organizations and NGOs. The health workforce in these countries had grown but remained thin. Liberia had only fifty-one doctors in the whole country. Guinea had one physician for every 10,000 people. Sierra Leone had 1,017 nurses and midwives total, one for every 5,319 people in the country. The average middle-income country has ten times as many doctors and nurses; wealthy countries have thirty-seven times more.

Hospitals in these West African nations lacked basic infection-control essentials like running water, surgical gowns, and gloves. Health workers were the first to contract Ebola and die from it, further weakening health systems and leading people to avoid health facilities and to try to treat their relatives at home. In the end, volunteer health workers and burial teams from these countries performed heroically in the crisis and, with the support of the US CDC, largely saved themselves. But the costs of limited health systems were high. Outside of West Africa, only one out of eight people treated for Ebola died because those patients received basic supportive care, including intravenous fluids for rehydrating. Inside West Africa, the case fatality rate from Ebola was 40 percent.

The international system intended to control outbreaks of infectious diseases failed miserably. For the World Health Organization, the Ebola outbreak was a debacle. Leadership failures, incompetent regional and country offices, and inadequate surveillance and response capabilities undermined the agency to the point that responsibility for the outbreak was given to a UN Mission for Ebola Emergency Response. Many countries ignored the International Health Regulations and imposed punitive and excessive trade and travel restrictions on West African nations. Jérôme Oberreit, the secretary general of Doctors Without Borders, said "it has become alarmingly evident that there is no functioning global response mechanism to a potential pandemic in countries with fragile health systems."[154]

Margaret Chan, the former Director-General of the World Health Organization, implored countries "to turn the 2014 Ebola crisis into an opportunity to build a stronger system to defend our collective global health security." Forty-five separate expert assessments were published about the Ebola crisis and their recommendations were largely the same: institutional reform and more funding for the World Health Organization, together with greater investment in epidemic and pandemic surveillance, preparedness, and response in poorer countries.[155]

Important measures have been undertaken to prepare for the next outbreak, most following the same script as past global health initiatives. A new initiative to develop vaccines for future epidemics is well organized and well funded, with support from the Bill and Melinda Gates Foundation, Wellcome Trust, and the governments of Norway, Japan, and Germany.[156] As of April 2017, twenty-one lower-income nations had participated in external evaluations of what they need to do to prevent human and animal disease outbreaks, but only three had begun implementing the results. After the Ebola outbreak, the United States dedicated $1 billion to help poor countries build the basic capabilities to prevent, detect, and respond to pandemic threats, but that important program is poised to expire in 2019 and US funding for pandemic preparedness will sink to its lowest level in a decade. The World Health Organization has been unable to attract much donor support for its new response system and the agency has yet to implement many of the deep institutional reforms recommended after the crisis.[157]

An outbreak of the Zika virus in 2015 provided an early test of this system and the apathetic global response bodes poorly for future global health emergencies.[158] Several years after the Ebola outbreak, coordination and funding of international epidemic and pandemic preparedness and response remain ad hoc and dependent on media attention. "We still are not ready for the big one," said Ron Klain, the former US Ebola czar, to the

Washington Post in October 2017. "We're frankly not ready for a medium-sized one. The threat is still out there."[159] Much of the opportunity that the Ebola crisis provided for enhancing global health security may have been squandered.

The Difference That Health Aid Makes

In recent years, an active debate has emerged over the effectiveness of foreign aid. The economist Bill Easterly and others have observed that substantial amounts of aid have not made countries like Haiti any less poor.[160] Foreign aid has also been criticized for making recipient nations the dependent, neo-colonial wards of donors (by economist Dambisa Moyo) or even propping up dictatorships (by Bill Easterly, again).[161] These are fair concerns and worthy of the debate they have received.

But viewed from ground level, in places like the Ethiopian countryside, the answer to the question of whether foreign aid has worked to improve health is simpler. Of course it has, and on infectious diseases, often spectacularly so. As figure 2.17 shows, every one of the diseases that international aid initiatives have targeted, from HIV/AIDS to malaria to newborn disorders, has declined dramatically in Ethiopia.

That progress against these infectious diseases has deeply reduced the number of deaths of Ethiopian children under the age of five. Those

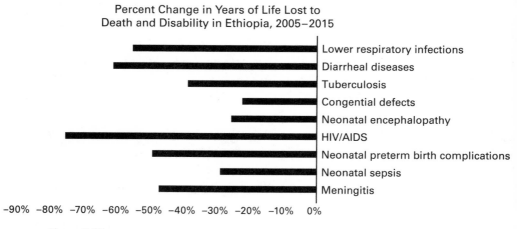

Figure 2.17
Data source: Institute for Health Metrics and Evaluation, GBD 2015.

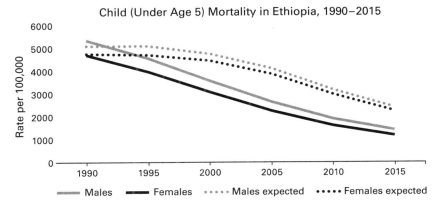

Figure 2.18
Data source: Institute for Health Metrics and Evaluation, GBD 2015.

reductions also happened much faster than would be expected based on the improvements in the country's level of income, education, and total fertility rate, as figure 2.18 demonstrates.

Most global health programs were not designed to establish primary care or public health systems, and they have succeeded in not establishing them. Many poorer countries have been slow to invest in their own health systems. That lack of investment in primary, preventative, and chronic health care in lower-income nations has left many of their citizens exposed to emerging threats like Ebola and the surge in everyday noncommunicable diseases. Greater dependence on donor-driven reductions in infectious diseases may also mean that these microbial threats are not playing the same role in forcing nations to invest in capable public health systems and responsive governments as these diseases did in the past.[162]

Inspired by the example of China, Ethiopia has hired and trained 38,000 community health workers to promote preventative health care in rural areas, which has improved child survival and lowered maternal deaths. The Ethiopian government, which is dominated by an ethnic minority group, has emphasized these community workers and the country's improved health performance as a way to build its national legitimacy and popular support.[163]

Nonetheless, so much of the recent health-related gains in Ethiopia was dependent on foreign aid. The country is the largest recipient of health and development aid in sub-Saharan Africa, at $3.9 billion per year.[164] Between 2012 and 2014, the United States spent $660 million on antiretroviral therapy and associated services for the 380,000 Ethiopians living with HIV. Between 2003 and 2009, Ethiopia also received roughly $3.2 billion in health support from the Global Fund and $70 million from the World Bank.[165] In contrast, Ethiopia spends less than 1 percent of its own domestic health budget on HIV.[166] Indeed, the Ethiopian government spends less overall on health per capita than its neighbors in the region.[167] Ethiopia devotes little of that small health budget to conditions that have not attracted donor attention. An independent assessment found that the country's health workforce suffers from a lack of professionalism and that doctors and nurses were so scarce in some hospitals that admitted patients often received care from their visiting relatives.[168]

The concerns over governance in Ethiopia extend beyond health. In a tragic echo of the past, Human Rights Watch accused the Ethiopian government of withholding donor-financed food relief as a way of punishing supporters of the rural opposition.[169] The government has responded to emerging protests in its large and fast-growing capital, Addis Ababa, by twice opening fire on protesters from the opposition party and rival ethnic groups. The government remains one of Africa's leading jailers of journalists. Ethiopian protestors disrupted World Health Organization meetings to decry the election of the country's former health minister to lead that organization. Ugly rumors circulated in the press that the Ethiopian government and its health ministry had hidden repeated outbreaks of cholera from international aid donors.[170]

Many donors and international agencies have justifiably been unwilling to wait for millions of vulnerable children to die needlessly from infectious disease in the hopes that the terrible toll might eventually inspire more responsive governments in poor nations. The Ethiopian government has emphasized that it is a young democracy and maintains that it is working hard to improve. So far, global health donors have stood by them.

Ethiopia may well emerge from its recent troubles with a more inclusive and tolerant government, but infectious disease is unlikely to be the catalyst for the needed reform. Ethiopia is not alone in this regard. Many of the other countries that have recently experienced faster than expected improvements in life expectancy, such as Rwanda, Zimbabwe, Nepal, and Niger, are also electoral autocracies dependent on heavy contributions of aid to achieve their health successes.[171] Rwandan President Paul Kagame, who was reelected in 2017 with 98.7 percent of the vote after eighteen years in office, has argued that the "true measure of democracy is not elections, but education, health, access to calories, and security for the people."[172]

History does not support that claim. Thomas Jefferson and a fellow signer of the Declaration of Independence, the physician Benjamin Rush, once argued that sick political systems and despotism produced sick people and disease.[173] The Nobel Prize–winning economist Amartya Sen famously argued, "Freedoms are not only the primary ends of development, they are also among its principal means."[174] Empirical research supports these assertions. In comparing countries of similar wealth, several studies have shown that use of social services and health outcomes like infant mortality have tended to be better in nations with free and fairly elected governments, with basic civil and human rights, and where people can make the spontaneous adaptations and innovations to public health systems that cannot possibly be planned by outsiders.[175] It is not hard, however, to think of counterexamples that have bucked the historical trend. Cuba has long maintained low child mortality rates and high life expectancy amid widespread poverty despite being a repressive, authoritarian state.[176] One must hope that Ethiopia and other recent global health success stories improve their governance, or at least prove to be sustained exceptions like Cuba has been.

Whatever the merits of that debate, it is evident that health has not been the bridge to popular support and legitimacy that it was for nineteenth-century governments or that governments in Ethiopia and other sub-Saharan African countries may have wanted. National surveys have also shown that six out of every ten respondents in the region report that they do not have access to high-quality health care, despite the dramatic declines in infectious disease in the country.[177]

Fortunately, there are other alternatives to letting infectious diseases and the other plagues of poverty run their course, or allowing donors to insert themselves between people and their governments. The conclusion of this book will consider a few other options for improving health while enhancing the role of social reformers and the local government. At the same time, the path pursued to dramatically reduce infectious diseases in Ethiopia and other poor nations has implications that go beyond health and unresponsive governance. The next chapter of this book explores diseases of childhood and the role they have played in the disparate fortunes of national economies.

3 Diseases of Childhood

The fatal and never-to-be forgotten year, 1759, when the Lord sent the destroying Angel to pass through this place, and removed many of our friends into eternity in a short space of time; not a house exempt, not a family spared of calamity. So dreadful was it, that it made every ear tingle, and every heart bleed; in which time I and my family was exercised with that dreadful disorder, the measles.

—Ephraim Harris, Fairfield, New Jersey, 1759[1]

Roald Dahl, the writer of *Charlie and the Chocolate Factory*, *James and the Giant Peach*, and other wonderful and often-dark children's stories, tragically lost his young daughter Olivia in November 1962. Nearly a quarter of a century later, he wrote the following passage explaining how it happened:

Olivia, my eldest daughter, caught measles when she was seven years old. As the illness took its usual course I can remember reading to her often in bed and not feeling particularly alarmed about it. Then one morning, when she was well on the road to recovery, I was sitting on her bed showing her how to fashion little animals out of coloured pipe-cleaners, and when it came to her turn to make one herself, I noticed that her fingers and her mind were not working together and she couldn't do anything. "Are you feeling all right?" I asked her. "I feel all sleepy," she said. In an hour, she was unconscious. In twelve hours she was dead.[2]

Olivia Dahl had succumbed to encephalopathy. This swelling of the brain, blindness, and deafness are the common and too-often severe complications of measles.

Measles is highly contagious and can be spread by the simple act of breathing near another person. Signs of measles infection begin with a cough, runny nose, and a rash of tiny red spots that starts at the head and spreads to the body. It then causes a fever. But the disease becomes deadly when its complications, like encephalopathy, arise.

Measles emerged from rinderpest (cattle plague) and began afflicting people as far back as fifteen hundred years ago. Because the disease was deadly to many, centuries passed before human populations grew large enough to sustain endemic measles, rather than occasional, fierce outbreaks that burned themselves out.[3] Along with smallpox, measles played handmaiden to the conquest and collapse of the Aztec and Inca empires in the sixteenth century. The same reason why measles was devastating to the Incas and Aztecs—lack of prior exposure—is also why it and other pediatric infectious diseases are disproportionately deadly to children like Olivia Dahl, who have not yet had and developed immunity to those diseases.

The first reports of measles in the American colonies began to appear in Boston and Connecticut in 1657.[4] Occasional outbreaks of it and other pediatric infections continued to occur over the next century and a half, but it was only with the decline of smallpox, for which there was a vaccine, and tuberculosis that diphtheria, mumps, scarlet fever, and measles rose in relative importance in the United States and Europe.[5] By 1900, respiratory diseases, such as measles, diphtheria, and whooping cough, took a heavy toll, collectively responsible for 28 percent of deaths of children under the age of 14.[6]

If you contracted measles in 1900, medicine could do nothing for you. The recommended course of action was basically to shut the door, isolate the child from others, and pray for God's good mercy. Measles is a virus, and the first human virus (yellow fever) would not be discovered until the following year.[7] The measles virus was isolated a half century later, when it was identified in the blood of a 13-year-old boy named David Edmonston. It was another nine years before an effective vaccine was developed in 1963. Maurice Hilleman and his colleagues at the drug company Merck released an improved version of that vaccine five years later and it now saves an estimated 1.5 million lives each year.[8] Before the invention and widespread use of that vaccine, 90 percent of American children experienced the measles virus by the age of 15.[9] Thousands of Americans each year were killed or left mentally impaired from the disease, usually as a result of encephalitis.

Effective vaccines were also developed for mumps and rubella in the 1960s. The widespread availability of these vaccines has improved children's lives so much in Western nations that their transformative benefits are sometimes taken for granted. A claim made by British gastroenterologist, Andrew Wakefield, that there is a link between autism and the mumps, measles, and rubella vaccine has spurred some parents to forgo vaccination for their children.[10] The study of 12 children has since been retracted by its publisher, the *Lancet*, but the claim persists on the internet and in the speeches of gullible politicians despite analysis after analysis debunking Wakefield's results, the decision to bar Wakefield from practicing medicine, and the reports that Wakefield had been paid by a plaintiff's lawyer to write the article.[11] As a result, the number of measles cases in the United States surged to 667 in 2014, a tenfold increase over 2010 when there were only 63. Fortunately, the number of measles cases in the United States has since declined.[12]

But the unfortunate resurgence of measles cases in the United States and a few other Western nations pales in comparison to the situation that until recently existed for children living in lower-income nations. Less than 5 percent of these children had access to the vaccines for measles and other deadly pediatric diseases in 1974.[13] Death rates from measles outbreaks in Africa were sometimes as high as 25 percent.[14] Five million children were dying needlessly each year from measles and other vaccine-preventable infectious diseases.

The success of the smallpox eradication campaign led some experts to believe that the same basic strategy could be extended and used against measles and other pediatric infectious diseases in poor nations. One person who was inspired was Jim Grant, appointed as Executive Director at the United Nations Children's Fund (UNICEF) in 1980. The effects of Grant's audacity and hard work over the next decade, along with the efforts of United Nations and World Health Organization colleagues and millions of vaccinators and health workers, still reverberate through the populations and economies of lower-income nations.

A Child Survival Revolution

UNICEF began life as the United Nations International Children's Emergency Fund—it later dropped the words "international" and "emergency" but kept the acronym. At first, UNICEF was a temporary initiative to provide clothing, powdered milk, and basic health care in the ruins of Europe after World War II. The agency later became a permanent part of the UN system in 1953 and expanded its services throughout the world, providing basic supplies and support for childbirth, feeding and nutrition programs, malaria eradication, and childhood vaccination.

In 1980, when Jim Grant arrived at UNICEF, it was a highly decentralized organization and most of its limited budget went to small-scale community programs to improve health and serve basic needs.[15] The international health community was focused on building primary health systems worldwide after the collapse of the malaria eradication program.

Grant was a World War II veteran, an attorney, and a former US aid officer. He spent his childhood in rural China where his father was a medical officer for the Rockefeller Foundation. According to colleagues, Grant was hard driving and not particularly sentimental about the sight of suffering children, but he believed passionately that it was possible to achieve progress in all settings, even those that were desperately poor.[16]

Grant was impressed by a report presented at a conference that argued that nearly half of all child deaths in the developing world were preventable at relatively low cost. "The road to health," wrote the paper's author, Jon Rohde, "does have short cuts." Vaccines existed to prevent measles, whooping cough, tetanus, and polio, which then killed roughly four to five million children each year. Inspired by that paper, Grant worked to overcome initial resistance at the World Health Organization to greater UNICEF involvement in childhood immunization. The World Health Organization had started its own Expanded Program on Immunization (EPI) in 1974, but it was reaching only 10 to 15 percent of the world's children and expanding slowly.[17]

Eventually an agreement was reached and UNICEF and the World Health Organization launched the Child Survival Revolution in 1982, with support from the World Bank and Rotary International. It was a staggeringly ambitious worldwide program, committing the organizations to more monitoring of children's growth; distributing oral rehydration solution to reduce diarrheal deaths; promoting breastfeeding; and immunizing 70 percent of the world's children in eight years against the six major pediatric infectious diseases: measles, mumps, tetanus, pertussis (whooping cough), diphtheria, and polio.[18] The program went by the acronym GOBI (growth monitoring, oral rehydration, breastfeeding, and immunization), and its goal was to cut in half the number of children who died worldwide.

The campaign began in 1984 in Bogotá, Colombia. For the rest of that decade, Jim Grant traveled the world armed with his props: a polio dropper, oral rehydration salts, and child growth charts. He met with heads of state, from military generals and democratic leaders, to rebel commanders and aging monarchs. He persuaded them to sign immunization pledges, allowing the campaign to occur and enlisting the aid of local officials. In El Salvador, conducting a vaccination campaign meant brokering a ceasefire in a fourteen-year-long bitter and bloody civil war for the sole purpose of immunizing children.[19]

Other NGOs and UN agency heads would not meet with the world's most murderous despots, men like Jean-Claude "Baby Doc" Duvalier of Haiti or Mengistu Haile Mariam of Ethiopia. But Grant would, and he convinced them that immunization would make them popular. Grant argued that UNI-CEF was in the business of "making a difference, not making a point."[20]

Even with the political support of local leaders and governments, the vaccination campaign remained a massive effort. It required building temperature-controlled supply chains in remote settings around the globe. It depended on millions of volunteers and the bravery of vaccinators who ventured into war-torn territories. Grant described it as the world's largest peacetime mobilization.[21] In 1990 alone, the program vaccinated 100 million children in one hundred and fifty nations six or more times.

The campaign met its goal and is estimated, in conjunction with the UNICEF programs on water and nutrition, to have saved the lives of

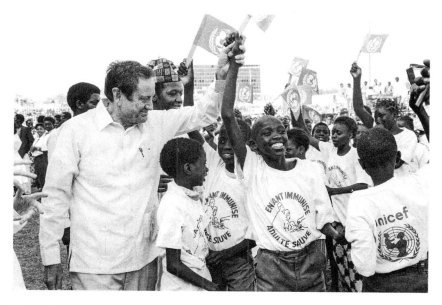

Figure 3.1
Jim Grant promoting child survival at Demba Diop National Stadium in Dakar, Senegal in 1987. Photo: UNICEF/John Isaac, Courtesy of UNICEF.

25 million children.[22] By 1990, there were only a dozen sub-Saharan African countries where as many as 175 children out of 1,000 still died before the age of five.[23] The rates of children fully immunized by their first birthday surpassed 80 percent in many lower-income nations, a rate that matched or exceeded coverage rates in some wealthy nations. It is an incredible story that too few people know, but that story does not end there.

International efforts to expand immunization for infectious diseases in low-income nations have continued and been taken up by others. By 1999, 470 million children under five years of age had been immunized.[24] In 2000, with support from the Bill and Melinda Gates Foundation and other donors, Gavi (initially the Global Alliance for Vaccines and Immunization) was launched to expand immunization programs to include newer vaccines for yellow fever, hepatitis B, and other diseases. Gavi programs operate in more than seventy countries, some with governments that are democratic and many that are not. From 2002 to late 2016, about $9 billion in donor funding, matching contributions, and cofinancing have been poured into Gavi. The return on that investment has been spectacular: 9 million children's lives saved since Gavi's inception.[25]

In the more than thirty years since the launch of the Child Survival Revolution, it has lived up to its name. Global vaccination coverage rates have never been higher than they are today; vaccination rates for measles, diphtheria, pertussis, tetanus, and tuberculosis in 2016 were all 85 percent or higher.[26] In the last fifteen years, for example, child deaths from measles fell 79 percent; expanded access to that vaccine alone has saved an estimated 20.3 million lives.[27] With the help of these pediatric vaccines and other global health initiatives, the number of children under five who die each year has dropped by nearly half—from 9.9 million to 5.9 million. Much remains that could be done to reduce unnecessary child deaths, but the progress first spurred by the Child Survival Revolution has been nothing short of amazing.

These spectacular health gains are reshaping the geography and age distribution of the world's population. That large demographic change offers a brief but important opportunity for poorer nations to lift their economic fortunes. But if that opportunity is not seized, the results could be deeply troublesome, especially in autocratic or fragile new democracies. To explain why, we need to go back to China in 1976.

China's Other Great Leap Forward

In 1976, China was among the poorest countries in the world. Its GDP per capita (measured in current US dollars) was lower than in Chad, Benin, or Niger.[28] The central government was in disarray after the death of Mao Zedong. Only fifteen years earlier, China had been ravaged by a famine that killed an estimated 36 million people, a famine that had been induced by the Great Leap Forward (1958–61), the government's disastrous attempt to catch the West by shifting the population from farming to making steel in backyard furnaces.[29] China was still in the grip of the "Great Proletarian Cultural Revolution," a political movement that included mass killings, shutting down schools, and exiling millions of educated young people to the countryside, including the current president of China, Xi Jinping.

The part of the remarkable story that everyone knows about China is that the world's most populous nation, after undertaking economic reforms in 1978, became one of the world's largest economies in less than forty years, lifting 560 million people out of extreme poverty and creating a sizable middle class.[30] What most people don't know is that China, by 1976, had already concluded a remarkable sixteen-year run in which its life expectancy rose a stunning twenty-one years. In 1960, the average newborn in China could expect to live only to 44.[31] A baby born in 1976, amid government-manufactured disasters and well before the subsequent economic boom, could expect to survive to 65.[32]

How is that possible? First, life expectancy, or more precisely the average expected life expectancy at birth, is a snapshot in time. Deaths that occur in the years past do not affect the expected longevity of a baby born later. Second, and more important for our story, life expectancy is also a lagging indicator of health gains that occurred in the past.

Between 1949 and 1978, China waged an all-out peasant-based war on infectious diseases, which dramatically cut its child mortality rate. In 1949, China adopted a three-year crash program to vaccinate its huge population against smallpox, and immunization initiatives against tuberculosis and diphtheria soon followed.[33] In 1952, the government launched the Patriotic Hygiene Campaign, a mass sanitation campaign that included latrine building, health education, and using chopsticks to pluck parasite-laden snails from ditches near villages.[34]

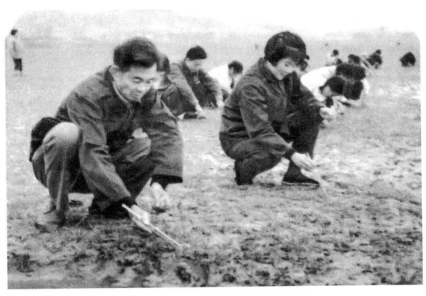

Figure 3.2
Contrary to this campaign photo, most of the tedious work of eliminating snails
with chopsticks was done by women and elderly, according to China scholar
Miriam Gross. Song wenshen: Huace (Beijing: Zhonggong zhongyang nanfang
shisan sheng, shi, qu xeufang lingdao xiaozu bangongshi, 1978), 65.

Beginning in the early 1950s, modestly trained medical aides were recruited
from village communes and charged with assisting clinic doctors to direct
rural hygiene and sanitation efforts and dispense antibiotics. They also
built thousands of clinics and health stations. In 1968, at the height of the
Cultural Revolution, this medical aid program was formalized and dubbed
"barefoot doctors" (*chijiao yisheng*). These barefoot doctors coached women
during their pregnancies, attended at childbirth, and educated mothers on
better care for their infants. They also collected so many stool samples, each
wrapped in paper or leaves with the patient's name written on them, that
some villagers began calling them "feces doctors."[35]

These stool samples were being tested as part of a national campaign
against schistosomiasis, a deadly parasitic liver disease also known as snail
fever. Mao was personally involved in the early planning of the effort. He
viewed the campaign as an important political initiative to demonstrate
that the Chinese Communist Party cared more for the people than had

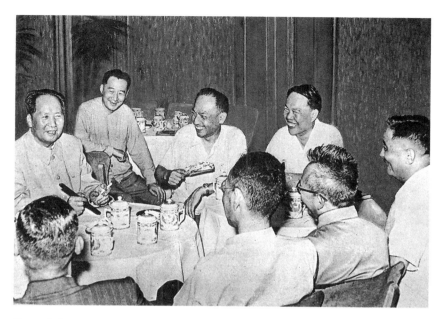

Figure 3.3
Mao (far left) consults with the Shanghai medical community on the snail fever campaign, June 1957. Song wenshen: Huace (Beijing: Zhonggong zhongyang nanfang shisan sheng, shi, qu xeufang lingdao xiaozu bangongshi, 1978), 11.

its predecessor, the National People's Party. Mao was reportedly so moved upon learning of the progress made against snail fever that he stayed up all night to pen a poem entitled "Farewell to the God of Plague." A whole generation in China was required to memorize and recite that poem from memory. Its closing stanza reads: "May I ask, God of Plague, / Where can you go? / Paper boats burn, / Candles ignite scorching the skies."[36] Mao's farewell to snail fever was premature; China still had fairly high rates of that disease and other infections such as tuberculosis in 1958.[37] Not all of the Chinese government's efforts to control infectious diseases worked; a public campaign in the late 1950s to exterminate "the four pests" (sparrows, rats, flies, and mosquitos) led to an explosive growth in the locust population and crop failures.[38] Even so, great progress had been made overall and, twenty years later, the children born in those years who might have died in the past had matured into working-age adults and helped remake China into a global economic power.

Is Healthier Wealthier?

It is tempting to cite China's spectacular economic gains that followed its improved life expectancy as proof that better health results in greater wealth. The empirical evidence for that theory, however, is mixed.

On one hand, there is intuitive appeal to the notion that healthier workers are more productive workers. The Nobel Prize–winning economic historian Robert Fogel estimated, based on changes in body size and calorie consumption, that better nutrition in the United Kingdom nearly doubled the labor output of working-age adults from 1780 to 1980.[39] Other studies have shown that hookworm infection and nutritional deficiencies have long-term effects on the wages and educational outcomes of children.[40] A commission organized by the *Lancet* and led by former US Treasury Secretary Larry Summers concluded that improvements in life expectancy in sub-Saharan Africa between 2000 and 2011 contributed 24 percent of the gains in "full income" of those countries, a measure that the commission defined as national income growth plus the value of lower mortality.[41] In 2015, 267 economists in forty-four countries, including Summers, signed a letter in the *New York Times* arguing that universal health coverage was "essential to eradicating extreme poverty."[42]

On the other hand, MIT economists Daron Acemoglu and Simon Johnson found in a multicountry study that income per capita declined slightly with life spans. This was because the economic improvement that resulted from higher life expectancy was relatively modest and had to be spread across a larger and growing population.[43] A study by economists Quamrul Ashraf, Ashley Lester, and David Weil concluded that raising life expectancy from 40 to 60 years would increase a country's GDP per capita by 15 percent over the long term, but only after enduring lower per capita income in the short run due to the economic "drag" of more children surviving.[44]

Given the many forces that affect an economy, it will always be difficult to isolate the effects of good health. But searching for a direct, mechanical relationship between declines in infectious disease and gains in future wealth is the wrong way to think about the potential contribution of good health to economic development. Jim Grant's Child Survival Revolution and Mao Zedong's peasant army of barefoot doctors are important in themselves for having reduced the deaths of millions of children. But they are also important for creating a golden opportunity, which, when paired with the right social and industrial policies, enables poor nations to lift themselves to greater economic heights.

The (Potential) Dividends of Demography

David Bloom, a professor at the Harvard School of Public Health, has spent his career thinking about how population and the economy interact. He and his colleagues have shown in several research studies that the relevant way to think about the role of population in spurring economic growth isn't size but age structure.

Nations with a disproportionate share of working-age adults, which Bloom defines as 15 to 64 years old, have an economic advantage. This demographic dividend, as he calls it, exists because that age structure means there are more potential workers to produce income and create things, with fewer dependents (children and the elderly) to consume them. While some readers might quibble with where Bloom and other demographers draw the line to define old or working age, China provides compelling evidence for Bloom's overall argument.

Starting in 1949, China dramatically reduced infectious disease and improved child survival, but its high birth rates did not initially fall. Mao promoted high birth rates and "national motherhood" in the early 1950s as a strategy to fuel economic and agricultural growth and possibly as a hedge against the threat of nuclear weapons and the deaths that would accompany their use. The Ministry of Health embraced birth planning in 1955, but the Great Famine and the Cultural Revolution interrupted the implementation of these programs. The birth rate declined in the mid-1950s, rose for most of the next decade, but started to fall sharply in the early 1970s. With more children surviving, Chinese mothers no longer needed to have so many of them. China also resorted to draconian measures to reduce its birth rate (which was already slowing), pushing women toward sterilization and brutally enforcing a one-child policy.[45] As many as a third of the tens of millions of people who died during China's Great Famine were infants.[46] The combination of these factors meant that more people born in the 1950s and mid-1960s survived into adulthood while fewer children followed in the subsequent decades. This resulted in a disproportionately large number of working-age adults, ready to take the low-wage manufacturing jobs that the 1978 economic reforms brought to China.

By 2000, people 15 to 64 years old represented more than two-thirds of the population in the East Asian region. Bloom and his coauthors estimate that one-third to one-half of the spectacular economic growth in China and other East Asian nations during this miraculous time can be attributed to the demographic dividend.[47] In a 1994 essay in *Foreign Affairs*, "The Myth of Asia's Miracle," economist and Nobel Laureate Paul Krugman also attributed much of the remarkable economic growth in the region to added inputs of labor, rather than a surge in productivity.[48] Similarly, the economist Robert Gordon argued that the dramatic decline in infant mortality between 1890 and 1950 is "one of the most important single facts in the history of American economic growth."[49] Most of the countries that achieved sustained economic booms over the last fifty years have had large and growing shares of working-age adults.[50]

For those lower-income nations now experiencing declines in infectious disease and gains in child survival, three lessons emerge from this research and the East Asian experience.

The first lesson, and the good news, is that rapid declines in infectious diseases, when paired with reduced fertility, can have an enormous impact on a country's economic development. Labor is a significant input to a nation's economy, and a large working-age population relative to children and retired people creates the possibility of much faster growth.[51]

Countries need not resort to the harsh measures employed by China to achieve this age structure. Japan, South Korea, and Singapore relied on voluntary measures to lower fertility in the 1950s. Overall, infant mortality rates fell from 181 per 1,000 live births in 1950 to 34 by 2000 in the East Asian region.[52] Better odds of child survival have generally been shown to substantially shape women's reproductive decisions, particularly in lower-income nations.[53]

Yet, while most East Asian countries experienced declines in infectious diseases, improved child survival rates, and reduced fertility in the 1950s, not all experienced the same economic gains from their demographic dividends. The economies of China, Taiwan, Singapore, and South Korea boomed. Thailand grew more slowly, and the Philippines grew even more slowly still. Outside the region, many Latin American and North African countries experienced only modest economic gains from their changing age structure.

These divergent results lead us to the second lesson from the East Asian demographic dividend: the demographic transition increases the importance of economic policy, magnifying the effects of good and bad policy choices.[54] As the share of the working-age population rises, the number of potential workers—the labor supply—expands. Good policies, sufficient investment, and dependable institutions are needed to create quality education, vocational training, and improved health, attributes that can make that increased labor supply more employable. Likewise, putting that growing labor supply to work effectively necessitates good roads, reliable electricity, rule of law, and sensible regulation that make it easier for factories to open and for entrepreneurs to start companies.

When these prudent policies are in place, a fast-increasing labor supply that results, in part, from a decline in infectious disease can dramatically boost the long-term growth of the economy.[55] The East Asian nations that reaped the rewards of their demographic dividend were able to do so because their governments combined a rapid demographic transition with targeted vocational training and export-oriented manufacturing policies. This increased the employability of their workforces and enabled them to take advantage of the growing demand to put all that labor to work.[56]

At the same time, China and these East Asian nations also got lucky, which leads to the third important lesson from the region's demographic dividend-fueled miracle. Without a supportive global economic and trading environment, the benefits from the demographic dividend would largely go to waste.

Make no mistake, China made many prudent decisions to capitalize on its declining burden of infectious disease. Joe Studwell, in his book *How Asia Works*, highlights three: the use of extension services to improve its agricultural yields; state support of entrepreneurs and technological upgrades to expand its manufacturing sector; and access to financing that targeted longer-term development and learning.[57] But it is also true that China lacked an open and predictable legal system, was subject to endemic corruption, and had a government that was not friendly to foreign investors. The average Chinese citizen had fewer years of schooling in 1978 than do the residents of most low-income countries today. Few would recommend that mix of policies and investments today for a nation looking to leverage its demographic dividend and grow into a great economic power.

China was fortunate, however, to enjoy its demographic dividend during a relatively egalitarian moment in the global economy.[58] In the early decades after World War II, Japan, Taiwan, and South Korea had to build a broad and deep industrial base to work their way up the ladder from making radios and other cheap consumer electronics to better-paid jobs producing sophisticated goods that could compete in the world economy. The invention of a standardized shipping container and lower tariffs changed all of that, allowing companies to outsource many more parts of the manufacturing process, sending the making of labor-intensive components and assembly of many consumer goods to low-wage manufacturers around the globe.[59] China, Vietnam, and other less-developed nations were able to put their demographic dividends to work and compete in the global economy through participation in these global supply chains, lifting hundreds of millions of their citizens out of abject poverty.[60]

Latin American nations were not so lucky. They too expanded access to childhood vaccinations and implemented better public health policies to reduce infectious disease rates.[61] Lower fertility rates eventually followed.[62] But these countries were mired in international and domestic debt, and suffered from high inflation. International lenders responded by demanding the adoption of greater budget discipline and fiscal austerity, adding to their economic woes and fostering cuts in education and health. Some countries, including Brazil, tried to respond by opening their economies to trade and outside investment, but were unable to create enough jobs for their fast-growing labor forces. Researchers attribute much of the stark economic inequality that still persists in Latin America to the failure to keep up with its changing demography.[63]

In short, a demographic dividend is not destiny. It is not a guarantee of economic growth. If, for example, the birth rate is slow to fall, then necessary investments in education are forgone because governments and families have fewer resources to spend per child. If economic reforms do not succeed and productive jobs are not generated, the number of working-age adults that are gainfully employed, and their incomes, will not rise.[64]

The window of opportunity that the demographic dividend grants is also relatively short. Countries that have recently reduced the burden of infectious disease and improved child survival must move quickly and forcefully. Governments, and donors that invested in achieving these health gains, should also invest in the necessary family planning policies to reduce population growth to sustainable rates and facilitate the economic and social reforms needed to take advantage of these favorable demographic conditions while they persist.

Is that likely to happen? We next to turn to Kenya, as a case example, to help assess the prospects for the future.

Sunny in Nairobi, with a Chance of Storms

Good things are happening in Kenya. For starters, its health situation, particularly in regard to infectious disease, has dramatically improved. Too many still die from HIV/AIDS, but the rate has fallen by two-thirds in just a decade. The great childhood plagues—diarrheal and lower-respiratory illnesses—are on the run, declining 27 and 21 percent, respectively, over that same time. Many more children under five survive than they did ten years ago, with Kenya's child mortality rates dropping by more than half to 12 per 1,000 boys and fewer than 10 per 1,000 girls. Primary school enrollment is up from 63 percent in 1999 to 86 percent in 2012. Average life expectancy has lengthened to 63 years for men and 68 years for women.[65]

Nairobi, the capital city, has become a hub for some of the world's biggest corporations seeking a foothold in Africa. It's a palpably multicultural city, with lots of people, intense traffic, countless construction cranes, and an accelerating influx of Western businesses. The *New York Times* travel section described the city as "surprisingly beautiful with flowering trees and the perfect climate: 70s and 80s, sunny, low humidity—almost every day."[66]

In 2010, Kenyans overwhelmingly approved a new constitution that is among the most inclusive in sub-Saharan Africa, with a strong bill of rights and more regional autonomy for the country's various ethnic groups.[67] The government is also making smart investments to improve its infrastructure and attract jobs. It is leveraging the seismically active Rift Valley to increase its geothermal energy output and electricity supply. The government is improving the road network and it has built a new railway.[68] Kenya has expanded its tax base to support those investments. More than 70 percent of Kenyans have a mobile phone subscription and nearly half have access to the internet.[69]

On the other hand, the demographics in Kenya are worrisome, especially given the structure of its economy. The population is growing very fast. It doubled over the last twenty-five years to about 40 million people, and that rapid rate of population growth is set to continue. Despite significant declines in child mortality, the fertility rate continues to hover above four births per woman.[70] Kenya's population is expected to grow by around one million per year—3,000 people added every day—over the next forty years and reach 85 million by 2050.

One of every five Kenyans is between the ages of 15 and 24. Its official youth unemployment rate is 18 percent, but the real number may well be higher. Less than 4 percent of Kenya's population is employed in manufacturing, and its exports, led by tea and coffee, have performed poorly in recent years. Kenya has an information technology sector, but its exports of that and other services have contracted in recent years.[71] According to the Pew Research Center, Kenya is one of just four African countries where the number of people living under $2 per day has increased significantly, from 22 percent in 2001 to 31 percent in 2011.[72]

More than a quarter of Kenya's people live in cites, a 29 percent increase in urbanization in just fifteen years. Nairobi's population has expanded from 120,000 in 1948 to 5.5 million in 2016.[73] The United Nations estimates that between 60 and 70 percent of those who live in Nairobi live in slums.[74] The share of the overall urban population in Kenya that lives in slums is 55 percent—a figure that did not change between 1990 and 2009.[75]

Kenya is entirely dependent on donor support for its supply of contraception and most of the medical treatment of its population living with HIV/AIDS.[76] The government is responsible for only $52 of the $204 spent on each Kenyan's health, with the remainder coming from foreign aid and out of the pockets of patients.[77] Meanwhile, deaths from cancer, heart disease, and other noncommunicable diseases are higher than the global average (624 versus 573 deaths per 100,000) and represent a significant share of hospital admissions.[78]

After independence, Kenya enjoyed relative calm, amid a far more turbulent and violent region.[79] In the past twenty-five years, however, almost every presidential race in Kenya has been marred by violence. In the 2008 election, 1,200 people were killed and half a million were displaced when ethnic rivalries boiled over. In the 2013 election, Human Rights Watch estimates that 477 were killed and 118,000 displaced. The lead-up to the most recent election in 2017 was ominous, with violent protests over government corruption and the discovery of the mutilated and tortured body of an election official charged with overseeing the vote.[80] Still, Kenya's donors had invested $24 million in an electronic vote-tallying system designed to keep the vote fair and free, and international observers from the African Union,

European Union, and the United States initially declared it so.[81] Around ninety deaths and dozens of sexual assaults occurred in the post-election turmoil.[82] In 2017, Kenya's Supreme Court nullified the result reelecting the sitting president Uhuru Kenyatta in an opinion that, over multiple hours, was read in full to a stunned nation on live television.[83] A later vote, marred by a boycott by the opposition, left president Kenyatta in office. Still, many saw the court decision to overturn the tainted vote and the comparatively less violent 2017 election as signs of uneasy, incremental progress.[84]

The situation in Kenya encapsulates much of what is happening in the rest of sub-Saharan Africa. There are so many positive trends. Infectious disease rates are declining everywhere. Between 1950 and 2010, the average years of completed school for adults in the region increased from 1.2 to 5.2 years.[85] Africa now has nearly twice as many cell phone subscribers as the United States. The contribution of remittances from the diaspora and foreign direct investment to Africa is about double the amount of foreign aid the region receives.[86] The economies of the East African region, which includes Kenya, grew at a healthy rate of 5.3 percent in 2016.[87]

But the demographic and employment trends in the region are daunting. Africa's population grew fourfold between 1960 and 2015, from about

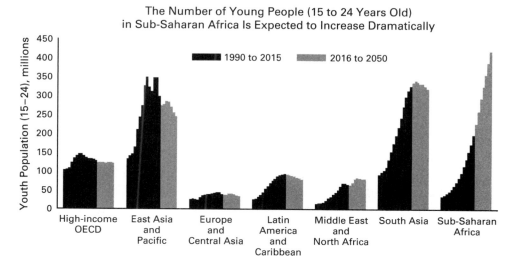

Figure 3.4

Data source: UN World Population Prospects. Adapted from: World Bank, *Youth Employment in Sub-Saharan Africa* (2014).

280 million to more than 1.2 billion people. It is the youngest of all the continents: an estimated 60 percent of its population is under the age of 24.[88]

More than half of those young people are unemployed or underemployed. Every year for the next ten years, eleven million young people in sub-Saharan Africa will join the job market.[89] This potential demographic dividend offers a tremendous opportunity for African nations to achieve a much-awaited economic transformation, but for that to occur, it will have to find a different path than the one taken by China or the nations of the West.

Cell Phones, Not Factories

For nearly two centuries, manufacturing has been the ladder on which the world's poor have climbed out of poverty. From the textile mills in Lancashire to the steel mills of Pittsburgh to the smartphone assemblers of Shenzhen, economic development has traditionally been led by manufacturing.

Manufacturing jobs have generally not required specialized education or skills and the wages tend to be higher compared to other sectors. That combination makes it easier for lower-skilled factory workers to advance themselves and their families into the middle-class. It has also been relatively easy to make and export low-end manufactured goods at scale, especially textiles, toys, or basic consumer electronics. Exports are an important source of foreign exchange and tax revenue, which are critical to developing economies. Manufacturing provides an incentive for governments to invest in building supportive infrastructure, such as roads and electrical grids, which have long-term economic benefits. South Korea and Taiwan are examples of countries that were able to start with low-end manufacturing, learn and invest in their workforce, and then move up to producing high-end manufactured goods and services and better-paid jobs.

Historically, manufacturing has also been labor-intensive: it employs a lot of people. That has been critical for nations confronting a fast-growing workforce of young adults.

A baby boom occurred in Europe and the United States after World War II. In the 1970s, manufacturing's share of employment rose to 27 percent in the United States and 40 percent in Germany. South Korea also put its demographic dividend to work in factories, and manufacturing came to represent 28 percent of overall employment.[90] All non-oil economies that became rich at one point employed at least 18 percent of their workforce in manufacturing, often before becoming wealthy.[91]

By contrast, manufacturing employment for lower-income nations is peaking at a far earlier point than it did for wealthier nations in the past, a process that Dani Rodrik, an economist at Harvard University, calls "premature deindustrialization."[92] This trend is a particular concern in sub-Saharan Africa. In 2010, only 7 percent of that region's workforce was employed in manufacturing, compared to 15 percent in Asia and 12 percent in Latin America. Manufacturing has represented the same share of overall economic output in sub-Saharan Africa since the 1960s. At the same time, agricultural employment in the region has fallen from 62 percent in 1990 to 51 percent in 2010.[93] Sub-Saharan Africans, like their counterparts in other regions, are moving from farms to cities. But they are not finding factory jobs when they arrive. Most of the private sector jobs created in sub-Saharan Africa over the last two decades have been in temporary or day labor. The government still provides most of the wage employment in the natural-resource-based economies in the region.[94]

Some of the reasons for the lack of manufacturing jobs in most countries in sub-Saharan Africa (and parts of South Asia) are the ones you might expect: too few roads and ports; too little power generation and electricity coverage; and too much corruption and labor regulation. But it also may be that the Child Survival Revolution arrived in these parts of the world too late.

Countries that are seeking to put their demographic dividend to work today face competition from low-wage manufacturing from China and the other nations who achieved those health gains earlier. Many sub-Saharan African manufacturers are overwhelmed by an onslaught of cheap imports from China, Vietnam, Bangladesh and other Asian exporters, which have greater economies of scale. That makes it difficult for sub-Saharan African manufacturers to survive on their home turf, let alone build an export-oriented industry.[95] China's labor costs are starting to rise, but that nation of nearly 1.4 billion people remains a formidable obstacle to new producers trying to build a domestic consumer base or make inroads into global markets.[96]

And then there are the robots. Manufacturing and many routine services have become increasingly automated. Factories can produce massive quantities of goods without having to hire as many laborers. Machines can also perform routine services, such as translation and call center jobs, cheaply and effectively.[97] As more of those jobs are automated, the low-wage advantage that sub-Saharan African and South Asian economies, with booming

youth populations, might have offered is undercut. The World Bank estimates that two-thirds or more of the workforces in Bangladesh, Nepal, and
Ethiopia are susceptible to automation.[98]

The rise of robots also highlights the importance of good-quality infrastructure. If low labor costs are not as important anymore, few corporations are going to incur added transportation costs to source their goods
from settings with long customs delays or poorly kept roads. Automation is
enabling the United States and other developed nations to "reshore" some
manufacturing back home.[99] Even China and India, which still have relatively low wages, are automating to stay globally competitive. China is the
world's largest employer of manufacturing robots.[100]

At the same time, the loss of manufacturing jobs in the United States and
Europe is exacerbating anti-immigration sentiment and encouraging calls
for protection from low-wage foreign competition. This environment is not
likely to be conducive to negotiations to lower trade barriers to African and
South Asian nations facing a labor boom.

The path that many countries took in the past—employing their
demographic dividend in manufacturing and exporting their way to the
middle-class—may be closing. One alternative is increasing employment
in the service sector, but here too there are limitations. Most service sector jobs require either a lot of specialized education—medical school, law
school, an accounting degree—or little education at all, such as for a retail
clerk. Employment in high-end services is not a near-term option for most
of the young adults entering the market in developing nations. Low-end
services that depend on personal interaction are more resistant to automation and can employ larger numbers, but they do not offer the same track
to rising incomes and the middle class that manufacturing does.

Services are also hard to export. Wealthy countries already have their
own low-wage retail workers, and many impose licensing requirements on
specialized services sectors like medicine or law, which limits foreign competition.[101] Given the prevailing attitude in high-income nations toward
trade liberalization, that situation is not likely to change. Tourism is a growth
industry for many developing countries, but it is not a large-scale employer.
Africa is a marginal player in the global trade in services. In 2012, Africa
accounted for only 2.2 percent of the world's total exports of services and
just 4 percent of the world's services imports. A World Bank report suggests
that those statistics do not capture the services that are informally traded

regionally, like hairdressing or accounting, but the numbers of people and jobs involved appear small.[102]

The management consulting firm McKinsey has enthusiastically argued that the emerging middle class in developing countries may become an engine of growth by creating a market for locally produced goods and services.[103] According to the Pew Research Center, the middle class in developing nations, defined as those making between $10 and $20 per day, has expanded by 385 million people between 2001 and 2011. But that growth occurred almost exclusively in China, South America, and Eastern Europe. While extreme poverty has declined, the middle classes in Southeast Asia and Africa—the places that have recently seen the greatest demographic changes—have hardly expanded at all.[104]

Too many young Africans and South Asians are unemployed, underemployed, or working in the "informal economy" as street vendors, home-based producers of garments or other goods, or in waste recycling. In most regions, a greater proportion of women than men are informally employed. Outside the agricultural sector, 82 percent of the workforce in South Asia

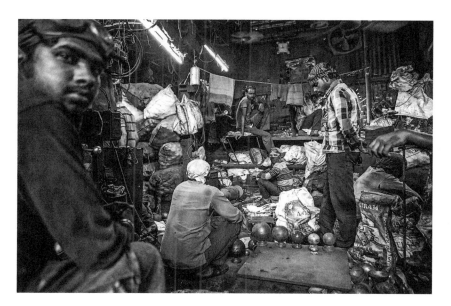

Figure 3.5
Informal industry in the Dharavi slum, Mumbai, 2016. Photo: Johnny Miller/Slum Scapes.

and 66 percent in sub-Saharan Africa are informally employed.[105] Informal sector jobs offer lower incomes and less security.

The economist Tyler Cowen predicts a different future for developing countries, which he calls a "cell phones instead of automobile factories" model of economic growth.[106] In his view, automation will lead to more centralized manufacturing in higher-income nations. This will mean fewer manufacturing jobs in poor nations. Cell phones, pharmaceuticals, consumer goods, and software will become extremely cheap and plentiful, but wages will stagnate and infrastructure will remain ramshackle. Nations that are close to advanced manufacturing countries, like Mexico, will benefit and be able to participate in those supply chains. Nations that are more remote might specialize in cultural production, computer programming, or information technology, as India has. Many other developing nations will be left on the sidelines of the world economy, with their employment dominated by informal or dead-end domestic service sectors offering little prospect of economic advancement.

This is a plausible future, but a deeply worrisome one for sub-Saharan African and South Asian nations facing large-scale demographic shifts and for the world as a whole. A failure to absorb a fast-growing, mostly unskilled labor force will have consequences in many developing countries that go beyond slower economic growth.

World Bank President Jim Kim has expressed concern about the convergence of aspirations that may come with widespread access to the internet, increasing the demand for the incomes and lifestyles of people in wealthy nations that youth in poorer countries see online. By 2022, three-quarters of a billion people in sub-Saharan Africa are projected to have smartphones connected to the internet; South Asia will have more than twice as many smartphone users as Africa.[107] Digitally inspired dreams of young people may spur entrepreneurship and drive economic growth. But without the opportunity to fulfill those heightened expectations, Kim fears, the aspirations of youth may curdle into frustration and strife, spurring conflict, extremism, and higher rates of migration.[108]

The Perils of Youth

Researchers refer to having a large proportion of adolescents and young adults as a "youth bulge." Those researchers favor different definitions of young adults, but it can range from 15 to 29 years old. Being born into a generation with a youth bulge can reduce young people's wages and increases the risk of large-scale unemployment.[109]

The region best known for its youth bulge is the Middle East and North Africa. The emergence of that bulge coincided with the collapse of oil prices in the mid-1980s, which undermined economic growth.[110] A fast-growing workforce resulted in high rates of unemployment, on average about 15 percent, which disproportionately affected young adults entering the labor market for the first time.[111] The youth unemployment rate was twice that of the overall labor force in a number of the region's countries.[112] Dissatisfaction, especially among educated youth, was high. In countries ranging from Syria to Tunisia to Egypt, it became a precursor to political and social instability and conflict.

A future of strife and violence is not the inevitable outcome of a youth bulge. Research by Colin Kahl, a political scientist at Stanford University, has found that the risks posed by a disproportionate number of young, underemployed adults increase only under certain circumstances: first, where strong collective religious and ethnic identities exist; second, when there are preexisting divisions between those groups; and third, when the state is too corrupt or weak to defuse growing tensions. Without that dry kindling, the evidence is weak that a youth bulge alone will lead to instability.[113]

Unfortunately, that dry kindling is in ample supply in many of the countries currently facing a youth bulge, including those in sub-Saharan Africa and South Asia, the regions that most recently experienced the greatest declines in infectious diseases and improvements in child survival. The World Bank estimates 200 million people in Africa are between the ages of 15 and 24 and that number is expected to roughly double by 2045. South Asia is also experiencing a youth bulge with an annual population growth rate of 1.2 percent. Two-thirds of the world's population growth in the next thirty years will occur in just fourteen large, lower-income nations: India, Pakistan, Nigeria, Indonesia, Bangladesh, Ethiopia, Democratic Republic of the Congo, the Philippines, Tanzania, Uganda, Sudan, Afghanistan, Iraq, and Kenya.[114]

Demography is now working against many of these countries.[115] Unemployment, particularly among Africa's growing youth population of 400 million, is a threat to inclusive development and social cohesion.[116] It is not hard to envision a scenario in which the next twenty years are even less peaceful than the last. That is bad news, not only because it could halt the recent impressive declines in poverty, but also because it could set back the very hopes for progress in poor settings that first motivated the heroic efforts in the Child Survival Revolution and subsequent global health programs.

There are alternatives. More investment in the economies and infrastructures of cities in developing countries could make a big difference. Urban areas have historically absorbed, housed, and employed the surplus of youth that followed declining rates of infectious diseases. We could also allow these governments to do what governments have long done when facing a population of young adults that outstrips the capacity of the labor market to absorb and productively employ them: let those people move abroad. The next two chapters address these possibilities—first, exploring the links between declining rates of infectious diseases and cities, and, next, moving on to the role of plagues and parasites in the migration of people.

4 Diseases of Settlement

Cities were once the most helpless and devastated victims of disease, but they became great disease conquerors.

—Jane Jacobs, *The Death and Life of Great American Cities*

In Dhaka, the capital city of Bangladesh, nearly 16 million people are crowded into 125 square miles. This is the equivalent of the combined populations of New York City, Los Angeles, and Chicago packing into an area the size of Greensboro, North Carolina, a quiet mid-sized US city with only 300,000 inhabitants. Most of Dhaka's residents seem to be stuck in the same traffic jam. The streets are a riot of rickshaw runners, cars, and "baby taxis" (motorized tricycles). The air is clogged with fumes and filled with the sounds of autos honking, laborers hammering, and the promises of restaurants and shops broadcast over loudspeakers. Parts of Dhaka have leafy green spaces, wide streets, and regularly emptied trashcans, but the southern sections of the city are not well maintained. The Buriganga River snakes through the city, black with waste from upriver tanneries and sewage treatment plants. More than a third of the city's population lives in slums, hand-built shanty-towns that line the riverbanks and the swampy lowlands, huddled in the shadows of hotels and high-rise offices. Dhaka is the most densely populated place on earth, swollen with people, promise, and peril.

Dhaka is an extreme example of two trends. First, it is a fast-growing city, which is a relatively recent phenomenon in human history. For ten thousand years, the share of the world's population that lived in urban areas grew very slowly. In 1800, only 3 percent of humanity resided in cities. In the nineteenth century, urbanization accelerated and expanded to 14 percent of the world's population. In 2008, the world, for the first time,

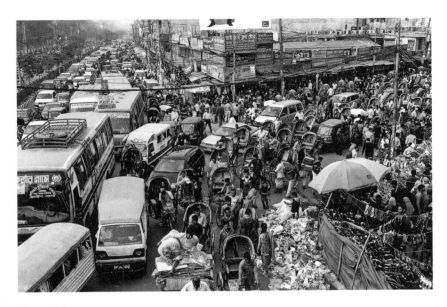

Figure 4.1
Traffic jam at a crowded street corner in central Dhaka, Bangladesh, February 3, 2017. Photo: Ruby Rascal.

became more urbanized than not, with more than half of all people living in cities and towns.

Second, Dhaka represents a shift in the geography and growth of cities to poorer nations, which has occurred only since the 1960s. Once, almost all urbanization happened in wealthy nations alone. Now, the population of city dwellers is projected to grow by 2.5 billion by 2050, with nearly 90 percent of that increase concentrated in lower-income nations in Asia and Africa. Some of that growth will occur in megacities like Dhaka, metropolises with ten million or more inhabitants. Most of the urbanization in developing countries, however, will be in cities with fewer than one million inhabitants.[1]

Cities in developing countries, or poor world cities, like Dhaka and New Delhi, are overwhelming to visitors, a chaotic experiment in improvised survival conducted at a staggering scale. But urbanization in lower-income nations is a potentially positive trend that could offer billions of people better access to jobs, health care, and a gateway to the world economy. The urbanization that is occurring in these nations, however, is also fraught with great risk, which is related to how these poorer countries are overcoming their burden of plagues and parasites.

The history of urbanization has been occupied with the struggle to control the infectious diseases that accompany large human settlements, but it has not been the same story everywhere. Cities in Europe and the United States first grew despite the poor health they offered to their residents. The economic opportunities available in those industrializing urban centers drew migrants that sustained these cities even with the staggering toll wrought by plagues and parasites. Over time, the cities in wealthy nations overcame the urban penalty of infectious disease through investments in sanitation, the creation of public health institutions, and the introduction of housing laws. For the more recent generation of poor world cities, the opposite has been true, with urbanization occurring ahead of factory job openings, better sewers, and public health reforms.

To illustrate this difference and its implications, our story takes us first to the soot-covered nineteenth-century tenements and factories of Manchester, New York, and London. We then visit the refugee camps of East Pakistan (now Bangladesh) in 1968, where we will learn about the discovery of two recent US medical school graduates that helped shift the geography of the world's cities.

Cholera and the White Death

For most of human history, cities were prone to famine and the plagues brought by invading armies and the passengers, both human and vermin, on trading ships and caravans. The last outbreak of the plague in Western Europe occurred in 1722. The disease most likely disappeared as a result of increased use of quarantine and isolation of infected households and communities (a practice known as *cordon sanitaire*).[2] A sustainable food supply for urban areas became possible in the seventeenth century with crop rotation and the swing plow, which was mass producible and easy to use. These agricultural innovations freed farm hands from the land of their ancestors and generated the extra food that the first industrializing towns needed to grow.[3]

At the dawn of the nineteenth century, the promise of jobs at higher incomes in busy textile mills and factories enticed workers and their families to leave the countryside and move to European and American cities. The living conditions that greeted these migrants were appalling. To accommodate the thousands of arriving workers and families, housing was constructed with great haste and greater carelessness. Buildings were flimsy and poorly ventilated, and most were unheated. If the lack of heat was not incentive enough to keep the windows closed in tenements (when windows existed), the smoke and soot from surrounding factories and coal-burning fireplaces provided the necessary deterrent.[4] In December 1873, for instance, London was covered for a week in a yellow fog so thick that it killed cows; people reported not being able to see their own feet.[5] Rudyard Kipling said of nineteenth-century Chicago: "Having seen it, I desire urgently never to see it again. Its air is dirt."[6]

The quality of water and sanitation in these cities was no better. Prior to the nineteenth century, human waste in cities piled up in cesspools and seeped into the surrounding earth.[7] The first public flush toilets were introduced in European and American cities around 1810, but they could not keep up with the growing urban population. New York City in 1856 had one toilet for every sixty-three residents.[8] Manchester, which quadrupled in size between 1800 and 1850, had fewer public latrines than ancient Rome.[9] Many of these early toilets remained connected to cesspools, which quickly became overwhelmed with the volume of use. Wastewater overflowed into streets and down open drains, spilling into the waterways. There, trash and sewage, along with animal and human bodies, floated in a toxic mix of pollutants from tanneries and butcheries, befouling the same rivers many cities relied on for their drinking water.[10] Friedrich Engels, the German philosopher and colleague of Karl Marx, described the river Irk in Manchester as "a coal-black stinking river full of filth and garbage." Dickens described London's Thames River as holding "the black contents of common sewers and the refuse of gut, glue, soap, and other nauseous manufactures: to say nothing of animal and vegetable offal of which the river is the sole receptacle."[11]

Cleanliness was considered a virtue in nineteenth-century America, but in practice, US cities left much to be desired. Thousands of pigs, goats, and dogs roamed the streets of New York City in the first half of that century, feeding on refuse and decomposing filth. (It was not just a New York phenomenon; stories of pigs knocking over city residents and invading their homes regularly appeared in US newspapers at the time.)[12] Midwestern city parks were effectively public hog pens. Oscar Wilde observed that the stench from the patrolling pigs in Kansas City was so overpowering that that it "made granite eyes weep."[13]

Pigs and goats weren't the only problem. New York was home to some 150,000 horses in the nineteenth century; the healthy ones produced as much as thirty pounds of manure per day, which was left on the streets to fester. The average horse survived just two years in the poisonous urban environments of the nineteenth century; thousands of horse carcasses were left on city streets each year.[14] Many city residents lived in tiny, unventilated apartments that often adjoined stables, factories, and slaughterhouses.[15] In 1832, a New York City physician reported arriving at 31 Renwick Street, a house in the now-fashionable Soho neighborhood, to find "forty to fifty hogs, four cows, and two horses." He refused to enter.[16] Piles of trash in New York City were often left in gutters, uncollected for days or weeks. New York City launched its first Board of Health in 1805, but it was staffed by aldermen without health expertise and had little authority.[17] Even when trash collection improved, New York City spent decades simply dumping the collected refuse directly into the ocean, including more than one million cartloads in 1886 alone.[18] Most American cities, and to a lesser extent those in Europe, had similarly deficient public health administration for much of the nineteenth century.[19]

The first large-scale urban water delivery system in the United States was designed by Benjamin Latrobe and completed in Philadelphia in 1815. Many US cities followed suit, often after years of haggling over water sources and how to tap and distribute them.[20] New York City chartered a company run by former US vice president Aaron Burr to supply the city with fresh, clean water, but that company (which later evolved into the bank JP Morgan Chase) routinely substituted poor quality water of dubious origin.[21] The first sewers in many American and European cities were designed to carry storm water and copious amounts of street waste flowed into them. The outlets of many of those sewers emptied upriver of the water intakes for city water systems. In 1827, for example, a Royal Commission in Britain found that several major companies drew the water they supplied to customers from the Thames directly across from the largest sewer outlet in London.[22] This produced in many American and European cities what David Cutler and Grant Miller have termed "circular water systems," where urban residents effectively drank water polluted with their own waste.[23]

Unsurprisingly, infectious diseases killed droves of the migrants who flocked to industrializing European and US cities. With larger numbers of people living and working together in confined spaces and sharing the

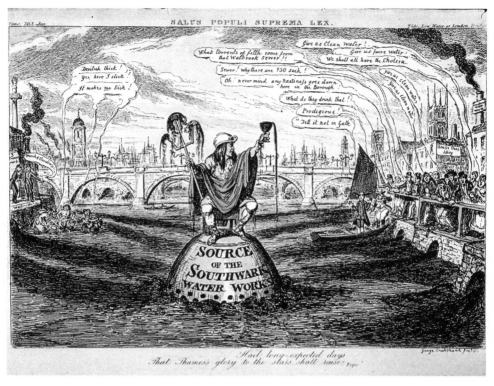

Figure 4.2
John Edwards, owner of the Southwark Water Works, depicted as Neptune in the
Thames River; with a chamber pot for a crown, a trident with dead river animals on
the prongs and sewage pouring in across from the water-intake. George Cruikshank,
Salus Populi Suprema Lex, 1832. Courtesy of the US National Library of Medicine.

same polluted water sources, the rates of respiratory and waterborne infectious diseases exploded.

The disease that did the greatest damage in these early industrializing cities was tuberculosis. It was not a new illness. Variants of tuberculosis appeared in East Africa as early as three million years ago, and the current strains are thousands of years old.[24] The disease is spread through secretions of the lungs and throat, which can occur with coughs, sneezing, and even breathing. Tuberculosis thrives in persistently impoverished communities and especially with prolonged exposure to the crowded conditions that characterized American and European cities in the nineteenth century. The most common form was pulmonary tuberculosis, a chronic form of the disease that became known as "consumption" in the English-speaking world. Tuberculosis can progressively destroy not only the lungs but also the central nervous, circulatory, lymphatic, and gastrointestinal systems and can scar bones and joints. Only about 10 percent of those who contracted the disease eventually developed active symptoms, but among those who did, four out of five died.[25] Tuberculosis was the leading cause of death (roughly one-quarter of all deaths) in industrialized nations in the nineteenth century. In its pulmonary form, the disease killed and disabled people of all ages, but disproportionately affected young adults. The historian F. B. Smith has said that tuberculosis "wrecked hopes, broke courtships, crushed breadwinners, and bereaved young families."[26] English churches hung the dried garlands and the yellowed white gloves of all the new brides who died from the disease. The terrible toll of the disease and the paleness it induced in sufferers earned tuberculosis the name the "White Death."

The poor working conditions in early factories facilitated the development and spread of tuberculosis.[27] Twelve-hour shifts and hot, overcrowded, and poorly ventilated rooms characterized most industries of this era, from textiles to metal grinding and glassmaking to bakeries and typesetting. Epidemics of tuberculosis followed the expansion of manufacturing in rapidly industrializing cities, first in Western Europe and North America, and later in Eastern Europe and parts of Asia.[28] In 1862, Engels and Marx grimly observed that "consumption and other lung diseases among working people are necessary conditions to the existence of capital."[29]

Tuberculosis, responsible for one out of every ten deaths in the United Kingdom in 1900, did enough damage to earn itself a literary following.[30] It cut short the lives of John Keats (1821, aged 25), Emily Brontë (1848, aged 30), Frédéric Chopin (1849, aged 39), D. H. Lawrence (1930, aged 44), George Orwell (1950, aged 46), and many others. The deaths of these young artists and other prominent victims inspired the archetype of the frail, pale, and beautiful protagonist dying too young of consumption that populates the poems of Shelley, the novels of Austin and Dickens, and the operas of Verdi and Puccini. The poet Lord Byron, who did not have tuberculosis, reportedly said he wished he would die of consumption so that "the ladies would all say, 'Look at that poor Byron, how interesting he looks in dying!'"[31] (Alas, Byron died prematurely from a different disease, now believed to have been malaria.)[32]

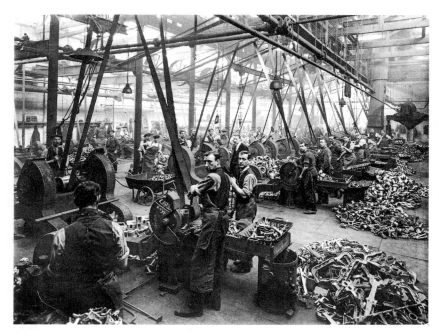

Figure 4.3
Men at work in a crowded metal grinding shop in Derby, England, 1928. Photo:
Leys Malleable Castings Company. Courtesy of the Derby Local and Family Studies
Library.

Cholera, on the other hand, inspired fewer romantic notions. The micro-
organism (*Cholera vibrio*) that causes the disease embeds itself with a hook-
like appendage in the human intestines and releases a toxin so virulent that
the body will discharge all of its fluids into the gut to try to flush it out. The
disease killed far fewer people than tuberculosis, but it attacked suddenly
and often publicly, causing vomiting, uncontrollable diarrhea, and, ultimately, severe dehydration. The terrifying disease struck seemingly healthy
people. The dramatic loss of fluids collapsed veins and turned skin blue,
drew victims' eyes back into their sockets, and could cause heart and organ
failure within hours.

Cholera was also not a new disease, but it had been confined to the warm
waters of the Bay of Bengal, which borders India, Sri Lanka, and Bangladesh.
With increased trade, the disease spread to cities in the Middle East, Europe,
Russia, and the United States aboard steamships and railways.[33] At least six

pandemics of cholera occurred in the nineteenth century. The pandemic in 1831–32 killed more than 20,000 in England and Wales and 3,515 in New York City (out of a population of 250,000). The next pandemic was even worse, with the dead numbering 50,000 in England and Wales and more than 5,000 in New York City.[34] While the death toll paled in comparison to the yearly losses of life from endemic cholera in India, it sparked rioting among the terrified citizens of industrializing Europe and America.[35] Crowded nineteenth-century cities, with rudimentary sanitation, poor hygiene, and few public health laws, were the perfect breeding ground for cholera, typhoid, and the other bacterial pathogens that pass from person to person through food and water contaminated by human waste.

The notion that urbanization extracts a penalty of poor health dates back to the late seventeenth century when John Graunt, an English haberdasher with a side interest in demography, began examining Bills of Mortality. English clergy began compiling these documents a century earlier to track deaths, births, and migrations and the practice spread countrywide. Graunt found that London recorded significantly more deaths than christenings and the 6,000 migrants that came each year from the countryside were needed to make up that shortfall.[36] The urban mortality rates in England and Wales, particularly from tuberculosis, were likewise much higher than the rural rates.[37] Charles Dickens wrote the following passage in a story about Victorian London:

> I saw a poisoned air, in which Life drooped. I saw Disease, arrayed in all its store of hideous aspects and appalling shapes, triumphant in every alley, by-way, court, back-street, and poor abode, in every place human beings congregated. ... I saw innumerable hosts foredoomed to darkness, dirt, pestilence, obscenity, misery, and early death.[38]

The urban health disadvantage that Graunt discovered dates back to the dawn of cities. Between the first and fifth centuries, the residents of Rome— slaves, freemen, and artisans alike—had lives about 25 percent shorter than their rural counterparts.[39] But the urban health disadvantages experienced in Europe and the United States throughout the mid-nineteenth century exceeded those seen in antiquity.[40] In 1863, the death rates in New York City, Boston, and Philadelphia were even higher than in London and Liverpool.[41] As late as 1900, life expectancy at birth was ten years greater in rural areas of the United States than in urban settings, and waterborne diseases accounted for nearly one-quarter of reported deaths from infectious diseases in major American cities.[42]

Despite the persistent ravages of tuberculosis and epidemics of cholera, migrants kept coming to American and European cities. During the 1849 cholera epidemic in New York, immigrants still came to the city at a rate of nearly 23,000 per month, enough to keep the factories staffed.[43] The unhealthiness of factories and cities, however, slowed the population growth of urban areas.[44] One reason was the appallingly low survival rate of children. A study in 1842 found that nearly two-thirds of deaths in London were of children under five.[45] Stockholm, Sweden, now known for its cradle-to-grave, government-funded health care, had one of the highest infant mortality rates in Europe during the 1850s.[46] In the 1870s and 1880s, the infant mortality rate in Hamburg was roughly ten times greater than the overall mortality of the city's population as a whole.[47] In the same time period, infant mortality was 140 percent higher in US cities than rural areas.[48]

Between 1850 and 1900, life expectancy in England and Wales increased by roughly six years and urban residents ceased being less healthy than their rural counterparts. Life expectancy at birth for males in New York City rose from 29 years in 1880 to 45 years in 1910.[49] Similar advances were seen elsewhere in Europe and the United States.[50] Japan followed with a 62 percent decline in its mortality rates between 1920 and 1937.[51]

The progress that led to these improvements was slow and occurred largely before the development of any effective medical treatments. In the case of tuberculosis, no one is entirely certain why mortality subsided. Louis Pasteur's discovery of pasteurization in 1865 helped cut the bovine form of tuberculosis that spread to milk-fed infants and children, especially in the US cities where it was adopted early.[52] The 1882 discovery by Robert Koch of the tubercle bacillus that causes tuberculosis gave scientific heft to already ongoing urban housing reform efforts. *How the Other Half Lives*, Jacob Riis's 1890 depiction of the infamous Gotham Court tenement, with Italian and Irish immigrants housed in crowded, tiny rooms without adequate heat, water, and sanitation, helped focus attention and mobilize reform. In Britain, legislation limited working hours, improved the conditions of factory shop floors, and mandated regular surprise inspections and piped water for residential housing.[53] Congestion eased somewhat in the more advanced cities, such as Paris and London. Better nutrition and immunity among the large number of survivors reduced the availability of new victims to transmit the disease. In the United States, local and national associations were organized and used catchy advertising campaigns to promote sanitary practices to control infectious disease, especially tuberculosis.[54]

Mortality rates from tuberculosis tumbled from their height of over 300 per 100,000 in 1840s England to below 100 in many industrialized nations by 1930.[55] Those rates fell further still with the modern era of tuberculosis treatment, which began with the development in 1921 of a partially effective vaccine, the Bacillus Calmette–Guérin (BCG) vaccine, and the discovery of streptomycin, an antibiotic, in 1944.

In the case of waterborne infectious diseases, acceptance of germ theory, public terror over cholera, and the slow building of effective sanitation and public health institutions made the difference. Repeated cholera outbreaks had demonstrated that selective sanitation only for the wealthy was insufficient to prevent waterborne disease.[56] The establishment of the first local and national boards of health in Britain followed. These boards, staffed with prominent social reformers such as Edwin Chadwick, used their new legal powers to begin to install water systems all over the country in the 1850s.[57] Their efforts to construct the accompanying sewers received an unexpected boost in 1858.

That year, an unusually warm summer produced such an overwhelming stench from the deeply polluted Thames that members of Parliament were overcome with nausea, an episode now known as the "Great Stink." William Budd, a prominent English physician at the time, described the situation:

> For the first time in the history of man, the sewage of nearly three millions of people had been brought to seethe and ferment under a burning sun, in one vast open cloaca lying in their midst. The result we all know. Stench so foul, we may well believe, had never before ascended to pollute this lower air. Never before, at least, had a stink risen to the height of an historic event.[58]

After every other effort failed, including dumping 250 tons of lime into the river to dispatch the stench, Parliament finally authorized the metropolitan authority to issue government bonds to pay for urban sewer systems.[59] Over the next two decades, roughly 83 miles of sewers were laid, supporting 100 square miles of the London area.[60] Tax rates rose to repay the costs of the investments in this infrastructure, but prosperity grew faster. The health (and olfactory) benefits of clean water and better sewage disposal were immediately obvious and not so expensive as to prove beyond the means of municipalities in other industrialized nations.[61]

In the United States, a similar pattern of political and social reforms unfolded, but more slowly. There was little or no sustained public health administration in the United States at the time of the first cholera outbreaks.[62] After an outbreak in 1866, New York City established the Metropolitan Board of Health, staffed by medical personnel.[63] Chicago, Milwaukee, Boston, and other large US cities followed shortly after.[64] Among the first acts undertaken by these new urban public health boards were banning roaming pigs and goats and forcing property owners to connect to the new waterworks and sewers being built.[65]

Fear of infectious diseases was one of several concerns that inspired the sanitation revolution outside Britain.[66] Industrial needs, fire protection, and rising consumer demands for the amenities of modern living were central to the creation of waterworks and sewage treatment in US and German cities.[67] But even in these settings, the threat of deadly infectious disease remained a powerful argument against those who opposed the taxpayer expense of piped water and sanitation and the frequent cost overruns in providing it.[68] The German city of Hamburg resisted investments in improved water and sanitation systems until a terrible outbreak of cholera convinced local leaders to reverse course.[69] With doubters silenced, other lagging European cities fell in line, investing in sanitation and better sewage systems. Widespread outbreaks of cholera on the continent have never returned. In Japan, investment in concerted public health information campaigns stressing hygiene and sanitation resulted in infant mortality rates rivaling those of England by the turn of the twentieth century.[70]

The number of municipal waterworks in the United States increased from 244 in 1870 to 9,850 in 1924.[71] Beyond expanding access to piped water, these waterworks also added filtration and chlorination, which remove bacteria like cholera and typhoid, larger protozoa like giardia, and most viruses. The percentage of urban American households supplied with filtered water grew from 0.3 percent in 1880 to 6.3 percent in 1900 to 42 percent by 1925 to 93 percent in 1940.[72] In 1857, no US city had a sanitary sewer system; by 1900, 80 percent of US city residents were served by one.[73] The improved access to filtered and chlorinated water alone accounted for nearly half of the decline in mortality in US cities between 1900 and 1936.[74] The

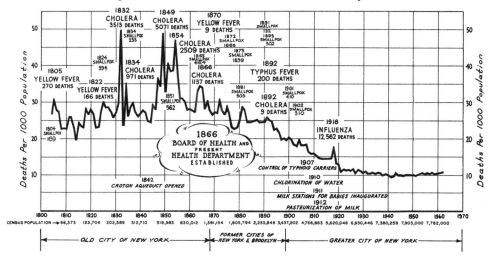

Figure 4.4

The Conquest of Pestilence, Summary of Vital Statistics, 1961, The City of New York. Reprinted with the permission of the New York City Department of Health & Mental Hygiene.

combination of public health reform, housing laws, and better sanitation dramatically cut infant mortality in Western European cities from 1850 to 1920. Clean, running water and indoor toilets also had the secondary benefits of enabling more manufacturing, improving the cleanliness of streets, and freeing women from the drudgery and time spent carrying fresh water into houses and apartments and dirty water out.[75]

As the historian Martin Melosi has pointed out, municipal governments were just emerging as effective institutions in the nineteenth century.[76] Building waterworks and sanitation systems was the first major undertaking for many city governments and the first that required significant financing, usually in the form of long-term loans and bonds. Many of the same strategies harnessed to provide clean water, roads, and effective sanitation to cities were used again to pave the way for later urban investments in intercity railways, ports, highways, canals, and education.[77] Popular referenda to mobilize public support for bond issues and repayment of past municipal debts made it easier to raise capital for future urban improvements. By the end of the nineteenth century, investment in city infrastructure was growing 4 percent annually in Germany and represented the majority of all government expenditure in the United States and Britain.[78]

With improved health and infrastructure, fewer of the people who moved to urban areas for economic rewards died; the population of those cities expanded and prospered. In 1854, less than 10 percent of the world's population lived in towns and cities of more than 20,000 residents.[79] In 1920, 14 percent of humankind lived in cities and nearly two-thirds of those urban dwellers resided in Europe and North America.[80]

The decline in infectious diseases and the gains in child survival that occurred in wealthy nations in the nineteenth and early twentieth centuries was only recently extended to low-income nations, where it has occurred in a different way that has yielded much faster rates of urban population growth.

A Simple Solution

In 1968, two American researchers were working on cholera treatments in Dhaka. Both were 26 years old. David Nalin had only just completed his first year of medical residency. Richard Cash had just finished his internship in surgery and had become a US Public Health Service Officer.[81] Their service in Bangladesh was done, in part, in lieu of serving in the Vietnam War.[82] The Pakistan Cholera Research Lab where Nalin and Cash served was established as part of the Cold War–era surge in US aid to Pakistan.[83] There, Nalin and Cash tested an oral solution of glucose and salt with twenty-nine patients, based on earlier scientific findings that sugar helps the gut absorb new fluid.

All of the patients treated were able to drink enough of the salt/sugar solution to survive. Those results set in motion the development of oral rehydration salts, which now cost a few cents per packet and have helped poor countries lower urban child mortality to rates that were once possible only with heavy investment in sanitation and public health.

Cholera and other diarrheal diseases have long been terrible killers of children in poor countries. During the late 1970s, World Health Organization officials estimated that there were about 500 million episodes of diarrhea in children under the age of five each year, resulting in at least five million deaths annually.[84] Part of the problem was that the standard of care at the time for extreme dehydration was saline provided intravenously. It was expensive, required the help of a nurse or physician, and was difficult to organize in infrastructure-poor settings. And, the circumstances in which Cash and Nalin worked were among the most infrastructure-poor and difficult in the world.

Bangladesh, then known as East Pakistan, was a destitute, densely populated, agrarian economy prone to frequent monsoons and floods.[85] The country lies in the delta of three rivers and most of its territory is only fifteen meters (fifty feet) above sea level. In 1968, Pakistan was divided by thousands of miles of Indian territory. West Pakistan kept most of the country's foreign aid for itself despite being wealthier, having more productive farms, and possessing a growing textile export industry. Seasonal outbreaks of cholera ravaged families and, occasionally, entire villages in the region of East Pakistan near its border with Burma. The research lab where Nalin and Cash worked needed to pick up sick patients in a speedboat—a five-hour journey—bring them back to the lab, and put them on intravenous drips, which otherwise would have been too costly or inaccessible for those patients.[86] The test that Nalin and Cash conducted in 1968 demonstrated that oral rehydration solution was safe and effective in treating adult cholera

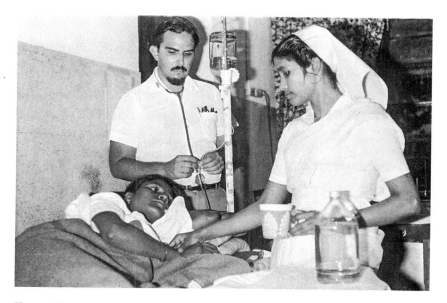

Figure 4.5
David Nalin examining a patient receiving IV rehydration, prior to starting oral rehydration therapy, 1968. (Courtesy of David Nalin.)

patients in an observed medical setting. They would later conduct further tests to show that the same was true for children.[87]

Three years later, in 1971, a civil war broke out for the independence of East Pakistan. Roughly 10 million refugees streamed across the border into India. Assigned to a West Bengal camp with 350,000 of these refugees, an Indian physician named Dilip Mahalanabis found that the supplies of intravenous fluid could not keep up with patients' needs. Mahalanabis instructed his staff to use oral rehydration solution instead and carefully tracked the results. Those findings demonstrated that oral rehydration solution was effective in responding to a cholera outbreak even outside a hospital or clinical setting. Nearly 4 percent of the patients that Mahalanabis treated died, but that was still an unprecedented improvement over the 30 percent who usually perished from cholera in those camps. Not only did the solution actually work, but it was more effective than intravenous fluids and could be used in emergency relief circumstances.[88]

There were plenty of opportunities for emergency relief over the next decade. Bangladesh's bloody war for independence was followed three years later by a famine that killed as many as 1.5 million people—2 percent of the population. The horror of that famine spurred a new generation of nongovernmental organizations (NGOs) to work with the government and foreign aid agencies to meet the health and subsistence needs of Bangladesh's deeply impoverished people.[89] In 1979, one of these NGOs, the Bangladesh Rural Advancement Committee (BRAC), began working with the lab where Nalin and Cash were stationed, later renamed the International Center for Diarrheal Disease Research, Bangladesh (ICDDR,B), to teach mothers to make the oral rehydration solution at home. This was no small feat, as many of the patients who would benefit the most from the treatment were desperately poor and mostly illiterate.[90] Starting in 1979, twelve hundred BRAC employees went door to door in rural Bangladesh and taught 12 million mothers how to make and use the life-saving salt solution.[91] That effort took ten years and, in more recent years, BRAC has extended the program to other poor nations.[92]

As a result of these collective efforts, oral rehydration solution—a cheap blend of salt, sugar, and water—has saved the lives of an estimated 50 million people worldwide, the vast majority of them children in poor nations.[93] The treatment has helped lower annual diarrheal deaths from five million to two million, despite a 65 percent increase in the world's population.

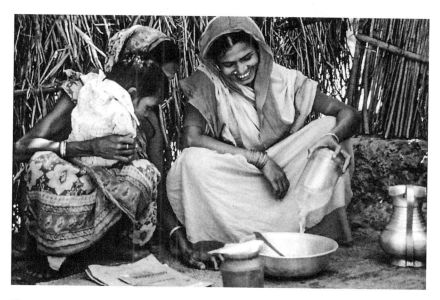

Figure 4.6
A villager learning how to make oral rehydration solution, Bangladesh, 1981.
(Courtesy of BRAC USA.)

More remains to be done, as roughly half of the world's children in developing countries still do not receive oral rehydration treatment.[94] Still, it is hard to disagree with the prestigious British medical journal the *Lancet*, which in 1978 called oral rehydration treatment "potentially the most important medical advance of the twentieth century."[95] In 2006, David Nalin, Dilip Mahalanabis, and Richard Cash received the prestigious Prince Mahidol Award from the Thai royal family for their lifesaving invention.

The results have been particularly impressive in reducing infant and child mortality in Bangladesh. More than 83 percent of the cases of diarrheal disease in the country receive the life-saving treatment, one of the highest rates in the world.[96] Despite ongoing water quality concerns, the combination of oral rehydration solution, antibiotics, childhood vaccines, and other effective, cheap global health interventions has cut child mortality (under five years old) to below 5 percent in Bangladesh.[97] Bangladesh is one of eighteen countries that experienced life expectancy gains greater than ten years between 1990 and 2013. Bangladeshi NGOs, like BRAC, have continued to use community-based approaches to tackle other health challenges such as childhood pneumonia, tuberculosis, and post-partum hemorrhage. Despite high levels of corruption and limited resources, these NGO-led initiatives have helped the country sustain substantial reductions in tuberculosis, cholera, typhoid, and other diarrheal diseases.[98] With many fewer children dying, mothers are giving birth to fewer of them. Fertility rates in Bangladesh have dropped from 6.6 births per woman in 1970 to 2.3 births per woman in 2013—a feat that Hans Rosling, the late-health data guru, called a miracle.[99] The country is still poor, but its economy has been growing steadily for twenty years.

The city and country in which Nalin and Cash began their research has been transformed. The population of Bangladesh has exploded from 100 million to 161 million. This is the equivalent of half of the population of the United States inhabiting a space that is the size of the state of Iowa. Dhaka is the most densely populated city on earth, nearly 70 percent more dense than Mumbai, the second densest city in the world. When Nalin and Cash were performing their work, ICDDR,B was on the undeveloped outskirts of Dhaka. Now it sits surrounded by the slums that radiate out from the city. Since 1968, the year when Nalin and Cash conducted their first test, the urban population of Bangladesh has grown almost thirteenfold, from 4 million to more than 55 million, according to data from the World Bank.[100] It is one of the fastest rates of large-scale urbanization in history and the infrastructure in the country's cities hasn't kept pace. Until 2016, Dhaka did not have a freeway; only 7 percent of its space is dedicated to paved roads.[101]

As spectacular as the growth of Dhaka has been, it is by no means the only city in lower-income countries that is expanding quickly without an adequate system of public works to support its population. Municipal water systems in many of these growing cities are older, poorly maintained, and suffer from low or intermittent water pressure, which reduces the effectiveness of chlorination.[102] Many cities in low-income countries supply water on a rotating basis for a limited number of hours at a time.[103] Moreover, urban water systems are also only effective in fighting waterborne disease when paired with street cleaning and well-functioning sewer systems, which many poor world cities lack.[104] Waste treatment plants are rare in Africa and Asia, and treat only 15 percent of municipal wastewater in Latin America.[105]

The available evidence suggests that oral rehydration solution, childhood vaccines, antibiotics, and other cheap health-care measures have helped developing country cities overcome the penalty that once came with urbanization. Deaths from cholera and other diarrheal illnesses in lower-income countries are generally decreasing much faster than the incidence of these diseases.[106] Recent data from India show similar results, adding to the evidence that much of the reduced urban mortality of these terrible killers of children is the result of treatment (oral rehydration and access to health care) rather than prevention (better sanitation and safer water).[107] UNICEF data confirm that oral rehydration solution has been distributed widely over the past fifteen years in the cities of the ten developing countries with most of the world's cases of cholera and other intestinal infectious diseases.[108]

The oral rehydration salts first pioneered by Nalin and Cash and distributed by Bangladesh's innovative NGOs have not only prevented millions of unnecessary and preventable deaths but have also been one of a handful of cheap, lifesaving interventions that have enabled cities in developing countries to grow beyond the limits of their poverty and infrastructure.[109] In doing so, these humble salts have assisted at the birth of a true anomaly in human history: poor world cities.

Poor World Cities

Most of the largest cities in the world today are now in poor countries and emerging economies. There are thirteen megacities with at least ten million inhabitants in nations that the World Bank defines as low- or lower middle-income. Those are: Dhaka; Ho Chi Minh City (Vietnam); Kinshasa (Democratic Republic of the Congo); Bangalore, Delhi, Mumbai, and Kolkata (India); Karachi and Lahore (Pakistan); Cairo (Egypt); Jakarta (Indonesia); Lagos (Nigeria); and Manila (Philippines).[110] And, more are coming as urbanization in sub-Saharan Africa and South Asia accelerates.

Poor world cities are a recent phenomenon. The large cities that existed before the Industrial Revolution were capitals of far-ranging empires, such as Rome, Constantinople, Beijing, and Baghdad. There were never more than a few at any one time.[111] At the dawn of the nineteenth century, big cities began to proliferate, but only in the most advanced countries. Cities like London, New York, and Paris were centers of manufacturing with comparatively high wages, which drew rural migrants. They also benefited from improving government institutions, which kept more of those migrants alive. In 1900, there were a few large cities in poorer nations, among them

Beijing and Istanbul, but those cities were still much smaller and growing more slowly than their wealthier counterparts. That situation remained
largely the same all the way through 1950, when only Kolkata and Shanghai breached the bottom half of top ten cities globally.

A decade later, the growth in cities started to shift to poorer nations. No
low-income country with a per capita income below $1,250 (all figures are
in 2005 dollars) was more than one-third urbanized in 1960; six nations
with per capita incomes between $1,500 and $2,500 reached that threshold, almost all in Latin America.[112] Over time, the level of wealth needed
to urbanize progressively declined and shifted toward South Asia and sub-
Saharan Africa. The population of the world's cities is expected to expand
by 1.48 billion people between 2000 and 2020; 1.35 billion of those new
urban dwellers will live in cities in less developed countries.[113]

Figure 4.7 shows that shift. The points correspond to the GDP per capita income level of countries when they first became more than one-third
urbanized. The size of the point reflects the size of the population of that
country at that time. The shading of the points corresponds to the geographic
region to which that country belongs. By 2016, fifty-seven of the poorest
countries had more than one-third of their populations living in cities. The
existence of large cities is, for the first time, no longer necessarily indicative
of prosperity or good governance.

Today's poor world cities are not just poor relative to contemporary Western cities. They are also poorer in real terms than the cities in developed
countries were when they first urbanized many years ago. When the United
Kingdom became one-third urbanized in 1861, the average income of its
citizens was around $5,000 (in 2005 dollars).[114] The United States became a
majority urban country in 1920 with a per capita income, in contemporary
terms, of about $7,500.[115] Most lower-income countries urbanizing today
are years or even decades away from reaching that level of prosperity.

Sub-Saharan Africa is the most dramatic example, urbanizing rapidly at
low levels of wealth. In 2013, the region was roughly 37 percent urbanized,
and income per capita was a little over $1,000, again in 2005 dollars. When
Latin America and the Caribbean reached 40 percent urbanization in 1950,
the average per capita income of nations was $1,860. The Middle East and
North Africa reached the threshold in 1968, when per capita income was
$1,800; East Asia and Pacific reached it in 1994, when per capita income
was $3,620.[116]

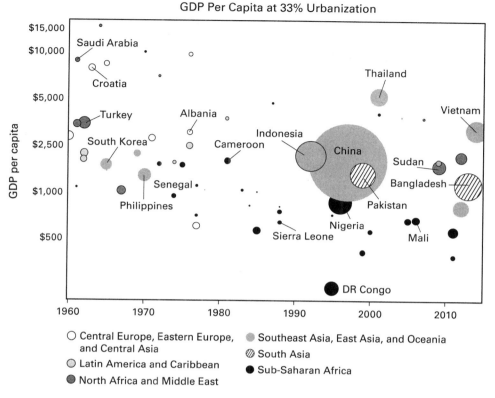

Figure 4.7

Data source: World Bank, World Development Indicators; UN World Urbanization Prospects.

Indeed, some of the fastest urban growth over the last sixty years has been in the world's poorest and worst-governed nations.[117] Most of today's thirteen poor world megacities are ten or more times larger than they were in 1950. They are also bigger than nearly any of the world's other cities were in 1950.[118] Only three of the world's ten largest urban areas in 2016 (listed in figure 4.8) are in wealthy nations with fairly well-developed public health systems.[119]

Not all of the urbanization that is happening in lower-income nations is confined to the crowded streets of poor world megacities either. Sixty percent of the urban population in developing regions lives in cities and towns with fewer than one million inhabitants.[120] These smaller cities are growing quickly too, particularly in South Asia and sub-Saharan Africa.

World's Largest Urban Areas, 2016

	Urban Area	2016 Population
1.	Tokyo-Yokohama, Japan	37,750,000
2.	Jakarta, Indonesia	31,320,000
3.	Delhi, India	25,735,000
4.	Seoul-Incheon, South Korea	23,575,000
5.	Manila, Philippines	22,930,000
6.	Mumbai, India	22,885,000
7.	Karachi, Pakistan	22,825,000
8.	Shanghai SHG-JS-ZJ, China	22,685,000
9.	New York (Metro Area), United States	20,685,000
10.	Sao Paulo, Brazil	20,605,000

Figure 4.8
Data source: *Demographia World Urban Areas* (2016).

So for the first time in history, cities are no longer restricted to wealthy and well-established nations. It is a trend that could have occurred only with the dramatic decline in infectious diseases and child mortality. But it is a trend that has not been met with equal enthusiasm by everyone.

Many visitors to the large, sprawling cities in lower-income nations find them congested, unattractive, and menacing. A cross-town drive in Manila or Cairo can take up half of your day. Thieves and aggressive touts selling wares might lurk in the park across the street from your hotel in Nairobi, the central square in Kathmandu, or the central business district in Johannesburg. Basic urban services, such as electricity, can still be inconsistent in many Indian cities. The geography of the sprawling slums and shantytowns in many developing country cities is not always intuitive to outsiders, popping up near the centers of the cities or shunted off alone under a highway overpass. A first-time visit to Delhi on "a hot stinking night" inspired Paul Ehrlich, a Stanford University biologist, to write his 1968 bestseller *The Population Bomb*, predicting overpopulation would result in mass starvation, environmental collapse, and the disappearance of England by the year 2000. Robert Kaplan's 1994 article in the *Atlantic*, entitled "The Coming Anarchy," sums up many of these concerns and may be the high-water mark, at least rhetorically, for Western alarm at poor world cities:

> I got a general sense of the future while driving from the airport to downtown Conakry, the capital of Guinea. The forty-five-minute journey in heavy traffic

was through one never-ending shantytown: a nightmarish Dickensian spectacle to which Dickens himself would never have given credence. The corrugated metal shacks and scabrous walls were coated with black slime. Stores were built out of rusted shipping containers, junked cars, and jumbles of wire mesh. The streets were one long puddle of floating garbage. Mosquitoes and flies were everywhere. Children, many of whom had protruding bellies, seemed as numerous as ants. When the tide went out, dead rats and the skeletons of cars were exposed on the mucky beach. In twenty-eight years Guinea's population will double if growth goes on at current rates.[121]

Concern regarding poor world cities is understandable. Atiq Rahman, a climate and migration researcher who leads the Bangladesh Centre for Advanced Studies, has called the explosive growth of poor world cities like Dhaka "a cluster of demographic chaos."[122] Overcrowding, pollution, poverty, and impossible demands for energy and water create an overwhelming sense that these swollen cities may collapse under the weight of their residents. But while concerns over the lived experience and sustainability of many poor world cities are well taken, there is reason to believe that some of the alarm at the phenomenon of poor world urbanization is wrong-headed.

Ed Glaeser, a Harvard economist and one of world's leading experts on cities, makes two convincing arguments on this point. His first point is that rich countries are urban countries.[123] No country has ever reached high income levels without urbanizing first.[124] Cities put people and resources in close proximity, which enables the exchange of ideas and the possibility of entrepreneurship. Cities also offer what economists refer to as agglomeration effects. These are the benefits that occur when more people are able to take advantage of the same public investment in water and sanitation, electrical grids, bridges and transportation infrastructure, or even health clinics. More people benefiting from the same investment lowers the per-person cost of that investment and amplifies its economic and social gains. Agglomeration is one of the key advantages that cities provide over rural areas and it has been sorely missed in many low-infrastructure developing nations.

Glaeser's second argument is an empirical one: the poverty in urban slums is bad, but rural poverty is almost always worse. The typical inhabitant in Karachi or Kinshasa may live in appalling circumstances by Western standards, but that person, on average, is still more educated, wealthier, and lives longer than the overall population in her or his respective country and has better access to essential services. Dhaka has lower rates of infant and child mortality than the national rates in Bangladesh.[125] Children's health in Korail and the other sprawling slums in Bangladesh is lamentable, but it is still better than that experienced by poor, rural kids.[126] As Glaeser writes, "while city-building is no guarantee of income growth, it has led to more prosperity more reliably than rural living in areas with poor soil quality."[127]

So may we chalk up poor world cities as a victory for the infectious disease control that will continue to improve? Not yet. We have very limited data on health in slums specifically; child mortality in Kenyan slums is improving, but the urban Kenyan poor are still less healthy than the rural poor, unlike in Bangladesh. There is more stunting and undernutrition in the children living in the slums of Bolivia and India than in the rural areas of those countries.[128] Poor world cities may yet be a potentially positive trend, but three aspects of the way that urbanization is unfolding should make us worry. Each has links to the way that infectious diseases have declined in many developing nations.

The Perils of Growing Naturally

Poor world cities have reversed the order by which urbanization has generally occurred in human history. When cities in wealthier nations were still rife with disease, the move from farm to town was appealing to migrants only if there were prospects for jobs in factories and mills at a sufficiently high wage to justify the risk.[129] The truly appalling sanitation and pollution and the high rates of deadly disease in those early cities kept the population gains from migration growing at a relatively slow pace. The only positive aspects of that otherwise unfortunate situation are the time it afforded countries to build wealth, an industrial base, and public health expertise, and the motivation it provided to some social reformers, political elites, and ordinary citizens for improving sanitation, roads, and governance.[130] This allowed the infrastructure and laws of American and European cities to slowly catch up to their growing numbers of residents.

As figure 4.9 illustrates, these trends are reversed in many poorer nations.[131] The economist Remi Jedwab and his colleagues have shown that much, if not most, of the population growth in many poor world cities is "natural," meaning that cities like Delhi, Lagos, Cairo, and Karachi are growing more because their residents are living longer and their kids are not dying unnecessarily, rather than because more people are migrating to those urban areas.[132] Child mortality is far too high in Bangladeshi slums—57 out of every

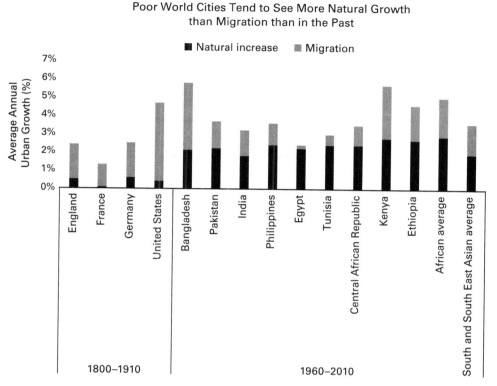

Figure 4.9
Data source: African Economic Outlook 2016. Adapted from Jedwab, Christiaensen, and Gindelsky, "Demography, Urbanization and Development: Rural Push, Urban Pull and…Urban Push?" 2015.

1,000 children under five perish. But that rate is still four to six times lower than it was in the nineteenth-century cities of the United States and Europe, where between 200 and 300 out of every 1,000 children under five died.

Indeed, as figure 4.10 shows, the poorer countries that have experienced the greatest and fastest urban growth have still enjoyed significant declines in deaths from the traditional diseases of density—tuberculosis and diarrheal and intestinal infectious diseases—that have long been deadly companions of city life.

Generally, mothers adjust to improvements in child survival by having fewer kids. With better infectious disease control and lower infant

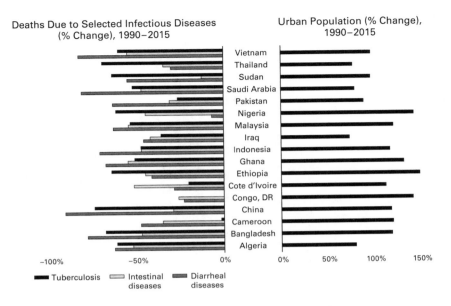

Deaths Due to Selected Infectious Diseases (% Change), 1990–2015

Urban Population (% Change), 1990–2015

Figure 4.10
Data sources: World Bank, World Development Indicators; Institute for Health Metrics and Evaluation, GBD 2015.

and child mortality, birth rates have fallen in the urban areas of lower-income nations.[133] Yet, in some countries, particularly parts of sub-Saharan Africa, the declines in fertility rates have been slow by historical standards, given the improvements in child survival in those regions.[134] As a consequence, the natural growth rate, which excludes migrants to the city, accounts for three-quarters of the overall increase in urbanization in Africa.[135] Part of the reason may be because fertility rates in slums tend to be high.[136] The lower rates of women's education in some South Asian and African nations may also be playing a role.[137]

Whatever the cause of the increase, poor world cities have been expanding at rates unseen in human history. Jedwab and Dietrich Vollrath estimate that London's fastest population growth, in the 1890s, was 93,000 new residents per year. The number of New Yorkers expanded annually by 220,000 in the 1920s. In comparison, Dhaka welcomed 445,000 new residents each year between 2000 and 2010, while Delhi added 620,000 people on average every year of that decade. The urban populations of Asia and Africa expanded as much between 1950 and 2010 as those in Europe between 1800 and 1910 in about half the time.[138]

Many poor world cities are making heroic efforts to keep pace with their fast-growing populations and to introduce the infrastructure improvements needed to support rapid economic growth. China has managed to build sufficiently productive cities to accommodate the waves of rural migrants drawn to its urban factories and to slowly improve public services.[139] Bangladesh, for example, boosted the share of its urbanites with access to improved sanitation from 47 percent in 1990 to 58 percent in 2015. That is a great achievement, but it was not enough. Given the spectacular growth of Bangladeshi cities, the number of urban dwellers living in that country without access to adequate sanitation (2.3 million in 2015) still more than doubled, from 1.1 million in 1990.[140] Population growth also outpaced the gains in access to clean water and sanitation in sub-Saharan African cities. The urban coverage of piped water in the region fell by 10 percent between 1990 and 2015, and only four out of ten new city residents arrived to find access to improved sanitation.[141] Similar effects can be seen in the provision of adequate urban housing, schools, and roads in many poor world cities.

Jedwab, Vollrath, and other economists argue that the high rates of natural growth and congestion in many poor world cities, if they persist, will overwhelm the economic benefits that cities typically offer through agglomeration.[142] In other words, the risk is that so many people may simply overwhelm the current urban water and sanitation systems, electrical grids, bridges, roads, and hospitals. In the last ten years, according to the World Bank, the average driving speed in Dhaka has dropped from 21 kilometers per hour to 6 kilometers an hour, little faster than walking. Congestion in Dhaka consumes 3.2 million working hours each day.[143] That reduces the utility of that infrastructure, which deters investment and depresses wages. If that pattern persists, poor world cities will be a historical anomaly in another way: they will be the first to keep their residents poor rather than make them richer.

One worrisome indication of that trend has been the expansion of slums. Overcrowded urban areas with informal housing, inadequate access to safe water and sanitation, and uncertain property rights are not new. Slums existed in eighteenth-century cities like Paris, New York, and London. Today's versions, however, are larger and growing much faster.[144] In 1910, the Lower East Side was the world's densest slum, with 140,000 people living in each square kilometer. Roughly 100,000 residents packed into each kilometer of Les Halles in Paris and the East End in London. The slums of Dhaka, Nairobi, and Mumbai have estimated densities of 200,000, 300,000, and 350,000 people per square kilometer, respectively.[145] The United Nations estimates 881 million people lived in slums in lower-income nations in 2014, which is roughly one out of every eight people alive that year.[146] The majority of those living in cities in Africa and Southern and Southeast Asia live in slums. In Kibera, the huge Kenyan slum in Nairobi, open sewer lines pour human waste in front of people's homes; hundreds of thousands of people share 1,000 public toilets.[147] In the Central African Republic, almost the entire country's urban population (96 percent) lives in slums.[148] In 2030, the population of slum dwellers globally is expected to number two billion.[149]

It would be easier to be hopeful for the long-term prospects of poor world cities if their residents were coming for the same factory jobs that provided a lifeline to more prosperity in other nations. Early factories in Europe, the United States, and China offered a hard life. They employed children, and workers labored long hours under deplorable conditions. Yet, as the economist Joan Robinson once wrote about underemployment in Southeast Asia, "the misery of being exploited by capitalists is nothing compared to the misery of not being exploited at all."[150]

Officials in many poor world cities are trying to increase their manufacturing base, but progress has been spotty at best.[151] Addis Ababa and the

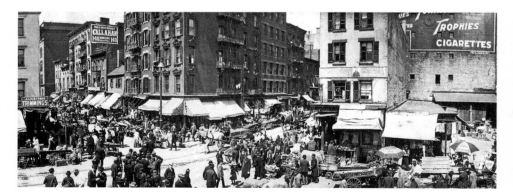

Figure 4.11
Hester Street, Lower East Side slum, New York City, 1902. Photo: Benjamin J. Falk, Courtesy of the Library of Congress.

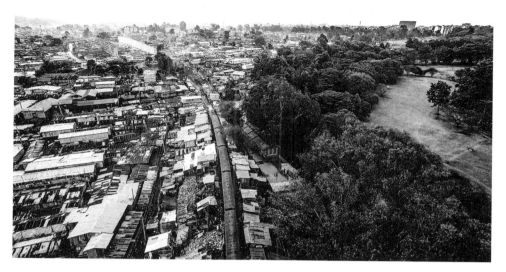

Figure 4.12
The Kibera slum sits directly adjacent to the Royal Nairobi Golf Club in Kenya, 2016. Photo: Johnny Miller/Unequal Scenes.

Ethiopian government, for example, are working hard to attract textile-manufacturing jobs. But those jobs may come mostly from Bangladesh, which has long occupied that same economic niche. Readymade garments account for 75 percent of Bangladesh's exports and are credited with increasing school enrollment and delaying marriage and childbirth among the millions of women who have been employed in that industry.[152] The garment industry is a major reason why Dhaka draws more migrants than most cities in lower-income nations. Still, the labor standards of Bangladeshi clothing factories justifiably generated worldwide concern with the terrible 2013 collapse of the Rana Plaza building, which killed 1,130 people and injured 2,500 others. The industry has rebounded since the disaster, mostly by cutting its already very low wages and prices to keep Western retailers buying, but hiring has slowed significantly.[153] But whatever its virtues and vices, the textile industry has not been large enough in Dhaka to keep pace with the growing number of citizens who need formal jobs. More than 84 percent of Dhaka residents are informally employed.[154]

The opportunities for formal employment are no more widespread in many other South Asian or African cities. According to a 2017 World Bank report, potential investors look at African cities and see crowded and disconnected areas with high costs for food, housing, and transport. The higher cost of urban living in many African cities requires local manufacturers to pay higher wages than in the cities of other developing countries. Africa's cities also suffer from a lack of adequate formal housing around the urban core. Consequently, people settle in relatively central informal settlements that are densely populated, ill served by urban infrastructure, and, by many measures, unlivable. Satellite towns also develop where land is cheaper, but the lack of paved roads and adequate transport services make it harder for residents to travel to capitalize on formal job openings that are more likely to be in the city center. This results in a paradox that many travelers to Africa's cities may recognize: they are sparsely built out and yet still feel crowded.[155]

Finally, the improvements in agricultural yields that traditionally enabled urbanization also have played a role in spurring the growth of the first poor world cities in Latin America and Asia.[156] But this has been less true with the more recent generation of poor cities. Improvements in agricultural productivity have not kept up with population growth in sub-Saharan Africa. International trade and aid has allowed cities, such as Port-au-Prince, the capital of Haiti, to compensate by importing the food that their growing populations need, an avenue that was not open when European and American cities industrialized.[157] This dependence on imported food leaves people in poor world cities vulnerable to world food price spikes.

The economic historian Paul Bairoch referred to poor world cities as "Romes without empires." As in ancient Rome, the rates of underemployment and unemployment in many poor world cities are high, and the food needed to sustain those urban areas comes from abroad. But, as Bairoch pointed out, there was only one Rome and, at its peak, it only had one million residents. There are now hundreds of poor world cities with more than one million people.[158] And many of these poor world cities are also contending with a changing climate and difficult environmental conditions.

Climate and the Environment

With great urbanization has come even greater pollution in many lower-income nations. Sixteen of the world's twenty most polluted cities are in South Asia.[159] Beijing's brown skies get most of the attention, but, as figure 4.13 shows, Delhi's air quality is now worse.[160] According to the Institute for Health Metrics and Evaluation, air pollution is the fourth-leading

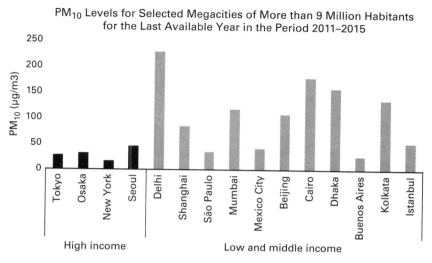

PM$_{10}$: Particulate matter of 10 microns or less

Figure 4.13
Data source: WHO Global Urban Ambient Air Pollution Database.

health risk globally, responsible for killing an estimated 6.5 million people in 2015.[161] Two million of them perished in India, with China not far behind. Poverty-stricken, crowded slums increase exposure to indoor pollution from cooking and burning fuels. To be sure, industrializing cities in Europe and America faced similar environmental challenges, but there is greater urgency in the current situation with the fast growth rates of poor world cities, the vulnerability of their slums, and the risks of spurring more rapid climate change.

Population pressures are also at work for poor world cities facing climate-related risks. Many cities are located along coasts or in river deltas, which had been beneficial for farming and commerce. But that historic advantage now exacerbates the danger to large, poor, and informally housed populations. These coastal cities need sea walls and other protective infrastructure to withstand extreme weather events, rising sea levels, and storm surges. That infrastructure is expensive and it will be difficult for many poor world cities to generate the necessary resources to cover the many people residing in their sprawling slums. A 2011 London School of Economics study found that nineteen of the twenty most populous cities exposed to coastal flooding are in poor and emerging economies. The only exception is Miami.[162]

These urban- and climate-related population pressures are at their most acute in Bangladesh, situated on a flat flood plain in the delta of three mighty rivers: the Brahamaputra, the Ganges, and the Meghna. Even the low-end estimate of a five-foot rise of ocean levels due to climate change would be disastrous for Bangladesh, forcing millions to flee their washed-away homes.[163]

Paradoxically, Dhaka, which is prone to flooding, is also running dry. Roughly 90 percent of the city's water supplies come from ground reserves, which are stretched to their limit. Dhaka suffers from a shortfall in its water of roughly 500 million liters per day, leading to angry protests over shortages in the summer months. Groundwater depletion is also causing the land underneath Dhaka to sink, which further raises the risk of flooding.[164]

If the dislocation that many fear from changing climate in Bangladesh occurs, one consequence may well be the re-creation of the refugee camps and regional instability that brought Nalin and Cash to conduct their cholera research so many years ago. But even before changing climate poses new tests, there are other ways that the rise of poor world cities might lead to greater conflict and instability.

The Tunis Effect

The populations of large cities, especially capitals, have long worried governments and despots. Urban uprisings produced the Roman Republic and started the French Revolution. Cities make it easier for people to assemble, share grievances, and find and mobilize other supporters for their cause. The wide boulevards of Washington, DC, where I live, are believed to have been designed by their architect Pierre L'Enfant to enable the military to more easily put down urban insurrection. Paris, in the nineteenth century, and modern Beijing were rebuilt with similar features.

The 2011 protests that began in Sidi Bouzid, a small city in Tunisia, over the self-immolation of Mohamed Bouazizi, a young unemployed university graduate, evolved into massive and deadly unrest when those protests reached Tunis, the capital city. A similar dynamic soon followed in Tahrir Square in Cairo, an enormous city, where residents protested against corruption, crumbling infrastructure, and state violence. Those protests toppled Hosni Mubarak, an aging dictator, and prevented him from installing his son, Gamal, as his successor.

The size, growth rate, and geography of poor world cities increase their likelihood of being hosts to instability, violence, and uprising in two ways.

First, the large slums in these cities enhance the potential for instability by having more people live in even closer proximity, making it easier to find like-minded compatriots even as the living conditions create additional grounds for dissatisfaction over overcrowding and corruption.[165] Poor world megacities have contributed to overall economic growth in each country, but they also have increased inequality among their residents, sharpening the contrast between rich and poor.[166]

Second, the rise of poor world cities has, in many cases, occurred in countries with autocratic governments. Cities are dangerous to dictatorships. Jeremy Wallace, a political scientist, has done compelling empirical research on 435 nondemocratic regimes in over one hundred countries, which shows that nondemocratic governments last longer in largely rural countries than in nations that are urbanizing.[167] In the most recent generation of poor world cities in sub-Saharan Africa and South Asia, those risks may be greater as rapid urbanization leads to overstressed infrastructure and increased visibility of corruption. Urban areas concentrate social stresses that might otherwise diffuse in rural communities, facilitating the forging of new political movements and ideologies.[168]

While the social and demographic pressures in many poor world cites may lead to messy and even violent disruptions, that may not necessarily be a bad thing in the long run. The links and social movements that form more readily in dense urban areas can ultimately force democratic reform and yield better government and institutions in countries where they have long been lacking. The social upheaval and protests in Western cities over the last two hundred and fifty years were sometimes painful, but they resulted in the institutions and laws that have been the foundation for progress on corruption, labor conditions, racial segregation, and, as we have seen, urban infectious disease. Economist and urban enthusiast Ed Glaeser calls this the Boston Effect, a reference to the role that cities played in fomenting the American Revolution.

But political upheaval and the sudden release of social stresses may not always yield better governments. Cities in disorder can also enhance the appeal of strongmen, who promise to tame the chaos and crime that comes with rapid urbanization. It is probably no accident that the Philippines, with one of the world's largest, most unwieldy and unequal poor world megacities, turned to someone like President Rodrigo Duterte. The former provincial mayor campaigned for office on the promise to use extrajudicial killings to stop urban crime and the drug trade.[169] The democratizing effects of cities, as Glaeser and his coauthor acknowledge, do not depend on wealth, but they are more likely to arise in places with a growing middle class. As the economist Nancy Birdsall has noted, Tunisia, which has one of the largest middle classes in the Middle East, not only started the chain of national protests that we now call the Arab Spring, but is the only one of those countries to have emerged "with something resembling democratic rule."[170]

Returning to Dhaka

The year 2016 was a time of upheaval for Dhaka and Bangladesh. On July 1, militants attacked the Holey Artisan Bakery, a restaurant in one of the Bangladeshi capital's wealthier neighborhoods, and took dozens hostage. Twenty-nine people eventually died, including eighteen foreign nationals and all five gunmen.[171] That attack came just a couple of years after several noted liberal bloggers, including one American citizen, were hacked to death by machete-wielding assailants in the city. Those attacks were reportedly committed in response to street protests calling for stiffer penalties for the country's wartime atrocities. The protests were started by liberal activists in the Shahbag neighborhood of Dhaka and involved more than 100,000 people.[172] The political unrest has taken its toll, slowing the growth of the garment industry, and may be deterring the investment that Bangladesh needs to advance beyond cheap, ready-made clothes.[173]

To be sure, the political unrest in Bangladesh has deep roots. Tensions between Islamists and secularists date back to the founding of the country, and the 2016 hostage crisis may have had ties to international terrorism.[174] Fringe extremist groups have a long history in Bangladesh.[175] The demographic pressure and rampant urbanization in Bangladesh and Dhaka have undoubtedly contributed, but it would be a stretch to link the country's recent political violence to the way in which diarrheal and other infectious diseases were reduced in this still-poor nation. It is fair to say, however, that the failure to move beyond NGO-led reforms contributed to poisonous Bangladeshi politics and ineffective governance. William B. Milam, former US ambassador to Pakistan and Bangladesh, has argued as much in the pages of the *New York Times*:

> Whichever [of the country's two main parties] was leading the government focused on enriching itself and weakening the other. That left the private sector largely alone to invest in economic expansion and NGOs to provide education,

health care and other social services the government wasn't delivering. In some respects, the government's failure to do its job served the country well: The economy has grown by an average of 5–6 percent annually over the last two decades; Bangladesh has outdone India and Pakistan on various social development indicators, such as health care and education. But the country's political culture steadily deteriorated.

Foreign aid has financed public investments in Bangladesh for decades, and a significant share of that aid flowed through NGOs, which were better able to deliver on their promises than the government.[176] The Bangladeshi government itself spends less per capita on health ($258) and still receives more of its health budget from foreign aid than most other South Asian nations.[177] The benefits produced through these programs greatly reduced human suffering, especially among children, and should be continued. But the failure to pair those programs against infectious disease with other reform-inducing measures has not helped the government prepare for the demographic changes that flowed from better health, including faster rates of urbanization.[178]

Alyssa Ayres, my colleague at the Council on Foreign Relations and a former US State Department official, has pointed out in US congressional testimony that the resources available to promote democracy and governance in Bangladesh have been quite small, especially when compared to heavy US assistance for health, food security, and climate change.[179] Investments in rule of law and better public institutions could help improve the human capital—everything from higher-quality education to a more rational and reliably enforced business regulatory environment—that fast-urbanizing countries like Bangladesh need to employ more of the young adults who live in poor world cities.

Without such investments, the job prospects facing many youth in Bangladesh and many other lower-income countries are still poor. As a result, many are seeking to move abroad in search of better opportunities. Bangladesh has one of the highest numbers of emigrants of any country in the world, 7.6 million in 2013.[180] The tie between that drive to migrate and the declining toll of parasites, viruses, and other plagues is the subject of the next chapter.

5   Diseases of Place

Time and time again I have seen NGOs and politicians in rich countries advocate that the poor follow a path that they, the rich, never have followed, nor are willing to follow.
—John Briscoe, Harvard University professor and leading authority on water resources[1]

Meningitis is a fearsome disease. Often difficult to diagnose, it causes the protective tissue around the spinal cord and brain to swell. You can go to sleep seemingly healthy and wake up deaf or paralyzed hours later, or worse, never wake up at all. If it goes untreated, its fatality rates can exceed 80 percent. It is a disease that disproportionately affects children and adolescents.

The *Neisseria meningitidis* bacteria that causes meningitis is spread through secretions of the nose and throat and extended close contact. In wealthy nations like the United States, small outbreaks of the disease sometimes occur on leafy college campuses, where it is passed by young people sneezing, sharing beer, or kissing. My sister contracted bacterial meningitis at her university and spent five terrifying days in a coma before finally emerging.

For unknown reasons, the most lethal type of meningitis, type A, is rarely seen in the United States. But it thrives in West Africa, where that strain of the disease surges with the harmattan winds that sweep through the Sahel, the transitional region between Africa's Sahara Desert to the north and its savannah plains to the south. These cold winter winds force people indoors, to huddle in overcrowded shelters. The arid climate dries out throats and makes it easier for bacteria to spread.

Researchers believe that Muslim pilgrims returning from the Hajj introduced type A meningitis to Africa more than a century ago.[2] Since 1905, epidemics of the disease have erupted every five to fourteen years in the "meningitis belt" countries—Mali, Niger, and the other twenty-three West and Central African nations where the disease is now endemic.

Over one million meningitis cases have been reported in Africa since 1988. A 1996 epidemic resulted in 25,000 deaths and over 250,000 cases, overwhelming already limited health systems and economies.[3] In 2006, affected households in Burkina Faso spent more than a third of their annual economic output on treating cases of meningitis.[4] In 2011, the average affected patient in Ghana lost twenty-nine days of work per case of the disease.[5]

Meningitis is a disease of place. Along with a dozen or so other parasitic, soil-transmitted, or bacterial infections, meningitis arises almost exclusively in the particular climates and ecologies where the world's poorest and most marginalized people live. Many of these diseases are known in global health circles as "neglected diseases," reflecting the lack of attention and funding historically devoted to them. That began to change about a decade ago, however, as the Bill and Melinda Gates Foundation, the US government, and other donors started spending between $500 million and $1 billion annually to develop effective drugs and vaccines for these terrible diseases.[6] Those efforts are bearing fruit.

In 2010, PATH, an international NGO working in global health, successfully developed a new vaccine against the type A strain of meningitis, working in partnership with the World Health Organization and with funding from the Gates Foundation. The Serum Institute of India manufactures the vaccine, which costs just $0.50 per dose and can remain effective for up to four days without refrigeration.[7] By the end of 2014, 215 million people in West and Central Africa had received the vaccine; not a single case of the disease has been reported among those immunized.[8] Cases of meningitis from the other strains of the disease, however, continue to occur and may be increasing.[9] Vaccines exist against these other meningitis strains, which are more prevalent in developed nations, but they are expensive. An affordable, heat-stable, combination vaccine is under development and expected in 2020. If all goes well, the goal of a meningitis-free Africa may soon be within reach.[10]

But progress does not stop with meningitis. A campaign led by the Carter Center has brought Guinea worm, another disease of place, to the verge of eradication. There were only twenty-two cases of the disease in 2016 in just two countries, progress that has occurred without the aid of a vaccine or medicine.[11] Deaths from African trypanosomiasis (sleeping sickness)

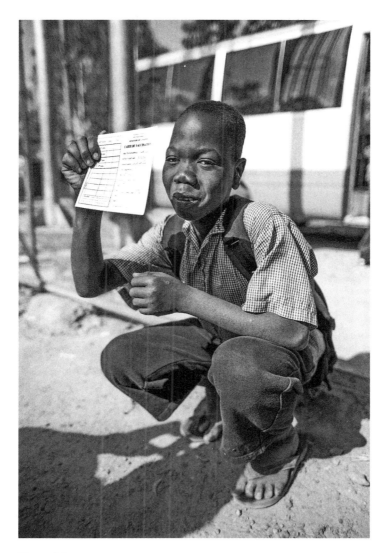

Figure 5.1
Boy holding meningitis vaccine immunization card in Burkina Faso,
2010. Photo: PATH/Gabe Bienczyck, Courtesy of PATH.

and leishmaniasis have likewise declined to several thousand each.[12] A new drug announced in 2018 for onchocerciasis (river blindness) may speed that disease toward elimination.[13] Vaccine candidates for other neglected diseases like shigella, another neglected disease, are in the pipeline.[14] Two days before Christmas 2016, the World Health Organization announced the successful completion of late stage trials of an effective vaccine against the Ebola virus.[15]

Many fear that the world's warming climate is becoming more hospitable to mosquitos and flies that spread neglected diseases that were once confined to particular geographic areas. The Zika virus spread in late 2013 from its historical confines in Africa into the Americas, where the virus was first detected in Brazil in May 2015. The reach of the disease has since extended throughout Latin America and the Caribbean, and as far north as the southern United States.[16] Zika gained international attention when it was linked to a surge in horrific birth defects in Brazil and other parts of Latin America. The concerns about the role of climate change in spreading Zika and other infectious diseases are another reason to ensure the continued success of international initiatives against meningitis and these other neglected infectious diseases. Those initiatives are bringing improved health and better child survival to even the most destitute corners of the world.

The Growth Industry in Agadez, Niger

If there is one country that illustrates the degree to which progress against infectious disease and child mortality is no longer dependent on income and the capacity of the state, it is Niger.

Not only is Niger among the poorest nations in the world, but its citizens are poorer now, with a GDP per capita of $363 in 2015, than they were thirty-five years earlier, in 1980, when Niger had a GDP per capita of $419 (all figures are in current US dollars).[17] A student in Niger may expect to receive five years of schooling, tied for the lowest amount of education in the world.[18] Just $71 is spent each year on the average Nigérien's health.[19] Niger ranks 101st in Transparency International's 2016 Corruption Perceptions Index, with a score that indicates a staggering level of public sector corruption. Niger is less than a decade removed from an armed insurrection in 2010 and it remains a weak state. Its neighbors to the north (Libya), south (Nigeria), and west (Mali) are themselves in the midst of violent insurgencies or are just emerging from them. Of the 188 countries that the United Nations ranked in its 2015 Human Development Index, Niger finished second to last.[20]

Yet, despite these difficult circumstances, a person born in Niger today can expect to live to be 61 years old, fourteen years longer than someone born in that country twenty-five years ago. Infant mortality has declined nearly 60 percent over that same time, to 57 deaths per 1,000 births in 2015. In just a decade, the death rate from HIV/AIDS dropped by almost two-thirds. Similar reductions were recorded in malnutrition (by 35 percent), malaria (by 27 percent), and diarrheal disease (by 48 percent) over that same ten-year period.[21] Overall, death and disability from infectious diseases in Niger has fallen by 17 percent since 1990.[22]

Unfortunately, even as child survival has improved, the birth rate in Niger has not declined. The average number of births per woman in Niger is the highest in the world, roughly the same today (7.3) as it was in 1980.[23] That high fertility rate may reflect the limited educational opportunities that exist in Niger for girls. But whatever the cause, it does not take a university degree in math to understand that more women each having the same number of babies on top of fewer of those babies dying equals a high and accelerating rate of population growth.

Indeed, Niger has one of the fastest rates of population increase in the world, 4 percent annually. Its population is projected to increase to 36 million by 2030, from about 19.9 million in 2015, according to the latest UN figures. At that point, the country will almost certainly have many more young adults than its economy can usefully put to work and even more children to support.[24]

To add to the county's challenges, as a result of climate change, the rainy season is becoming even less predictable in already drought-prone Niger. Eighty percent of Niger is desert, and most of it is uninhabitable. The combination of fickle rains and hotter days makes it even harder for Niger's farmers and pastoralists to produce enough food to make a living, precisely at the moment when it is most needed to support the country's booming population. Niger is losing arable land to desertification at a rate of 386 square miles per year.[25] Some of those farmers and herders are moving to Niger's cities, but they are finding job opportunities to be scarce.[26]

Given this set of circumstances, young Nigériens are doing what you or I might do: they are leaving, or at least trying to. Those young people who have stayed behind are increasingly employed in the business of helping their compatriots and the citizens of neighboring nations emigrate.

Once, great caravans connected through Niger's cities on their way to the souks of North Africa and the markets of Europe. But with the invention of shipping containers and the subsequent increase in seafaring trade, that caravan trade disappeared, leaving the city hubs of that trade destitute and forgotten.[27] Agadez, a small city on the southern outskirts of the Sahara Desert, was one of those hubs. Today, migration is the main business in Agadez, and business is booming.

In 2016, as many as 3,000 migrants passed through Agadez each week on their way to Sehba in Libya.[28] From there, migrants make their way to varying places along Libya's 1,770 kilometer coast, the longest of any country bordering the Mediterranean. Small boats leave for Italy under the cover of darkness, dinghies that drift amid the glowing oil platforms in the Mediterranean Sea.[29] About 170,000 people used the route through Agadez in 2015 and 150,000 in 2014. In 2016, that number grew to 311,000.[30] Nearly nine out of ten traveling the route are young men.[31] Nigériens and Nigerians comprised most of these migrants traveling through Agadez, with the remainder from Mali, Senegal, and Cote d'Ivoire, among other nations.[32]

After Agadez, the route for migrants becomes treacherous. Armed gangs in Libya are known to imprison migrants to extort payments from relatives. Women are particularly vulnerable; many are sexually assaulted along the route, often multiple times. Some are forced into prostitution. The risks do not end for those who make it onto one of the ramshackle boats that leave the Libyan coast for Italy. Nearly 8,000 people died trying to cross the Central Mediterranean in 2016 alone. The identity of most of those bodies cannot be determined, but the majority of those that could be identified were African.[33] Migrants have taken to writing phone numbers on their clothes in case their bodies wash up on shore.[34] According to the International Organization on Migration, more than half of the 80,000 migrants who made it to Italy's southernmost island, Lampedusa, in 2014 passed through Agadez.[35] Between 2014 and 2016, nearly half a million people arrived in Italy on boats from Libya, mainly from sub-Saharan Africa.

In their book *Migrant, Refugee, Smuggler, Savior*, Peter Tinti and Tuesday Reitano describe Agadez as a city transformed, with new housing, restaurants, fresh produce, and shops. A *New York Times* article quotes an Agadez deputy major, who states, "Many are eating off these migrants—the drivers,

The Central Mediterranean Migration Route

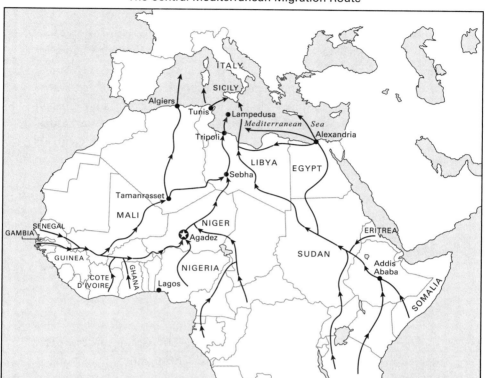

Figure 5.2
Adapted from UNICEF, *A Deadly Journey for Children* (2017).

the fixers, the landlords. The police are eating, too."[36] Reuters reported that Niger's security forces make a half million CFA francs ($850) from every round trip by a smuggling truck, not including the payoffs those security forces receive from gangs.[37]

Given the economic incentives and lack of viable alternative employment, migration through Niger will be difficult to stop. Further, most of the migrants who pass through Niger do so legally. Niger is part of a fifteen-nation bloc, the Economic Community of West African States, which permits freedom of movement to the citizens of its member states.[38]

Nevertheless, Germany, Italy, and other European nations are determined to reduce the numbers of migrants from Africa. In 2015, Niger's President

Mahamadou Issoufou requested a "Marshall Plan" for Niger to stop the flow of migrants and help reduce fertility rates.[39] European nations have responded, promising more than two billion euros in aid to improve security and economic development in that region.[40] A 2016 visit by German Chancellor Angela Merkel to Niger sparked a local crackdown that has shifted smugglers away from Agadez to more dangerous, less familiar desert routes. Stories of the skeletons of dead migrants littering these desert routes have begun to appear in Western media.[41] Talks between African and European leaders continue, as do efforts to tighten border control and asylum requirements and to return and resettle more migrants. In addition to Niger, the European Commission is also seeking resettlement agreements with Nigeria, Mali, Senegal, and Ethiopia—countries that, like Niger, have booming populations but limited, poorly paid job prospects.[42]

A century ago, European nations were on the other side of a similar combination of demographic forces, pushing tens of millions of their young adults to emigrate abroad. Ireland was at the forefront of that emigration.

People, Not Just Potatoes

In many ways, the great Irish emigration of the late nineteenth century is the closest precursor to the demographic-fueled migration happening in many lower-income nations today.

As in many developing countries today, the declines in infectious disease and child mortality in Ireland predated its industrialization, occurring when it was one of the poorest nations in Europe. Around 1780, a shift in agricultural practices toward tillage improved crop yields, particularly for potatoes.[43] Demand for food in England led to the conversion of pastures to cultivated land.[44] With more nutrition, the population grew, but the country did not industrialize like some of its neighbors. Ireland struggled to compete with the larger factories of England and the barriers that English industrialists had erected against imports of Irish goods. And so, Ireland remained mainly rural and poor, with most of its citizens trapped in the dreary, precarious life of tenant farming.[45]

Still, for all the poverty in the Irish countryside, in the mid-nineteenth century, a tenant farmer in Ireland lived a healthier and longer life than a resident of the smoke-choked cities of England, Wales, and Scotland, where infectious diseases remained abundant and continued to kill many children. The fertility rate declined in Ireland, but not fast enough to keep the population from growing quickly. By 1845, the number of inhabitants on the island of Ireland expanded to 8,525,000.[46]

When I was in elementary school, we learned that it was the terrible potato famine, which struck Ireland between 1845 and 1849, that pushed thousands of Irish men and women to leave their farms for the cities and seaports of America. In fact, young Irish adults began putting down their hoes and moving well before that. In 1821, emigration from Ireland to the United States was already occurring at a clip of roughly 13,000 people per year. The rate of migration rose to 93,000 in 1842, three years before the potato famine would temporarily double that rate. Most who left were 20 to 35 years old and disproportionately male.[47]

Irish migrants may have left for a better life, but they did not receive a healthier one. Mortality rates generally increased for the Irish upon leaving their homeland. Typhus and undernutrition were so rampant on the over-crowded voyages to the United States that they became known as coffin ships.[48] Upon arrival in New York, Boston, and other US cities, many of the

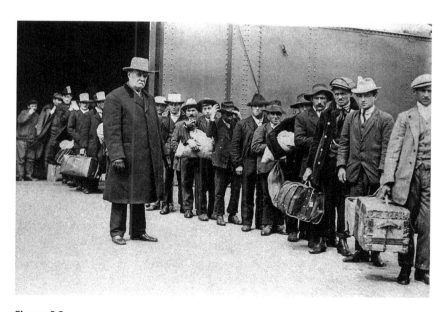

Figure 5.3
Immigrants from Ireland waiting in line at Ellis Island, 1911. Photo: CORBIS/Getty Images.

Irish migrants who survived found shelter in tenements that were poorly ventilated, overstuffed with residents, and rife with tuberculosis.

Between 1850 and 1913, an average of 13,000 young men and women emigrated from Ireland every year.[49] Among those migrants were John Cashman, age 18, and Alicia Dowling, age 17. They later met in Bayonne, New Jersey, married, and had a son who became the grandfather to my wife (I am forever grateful for John and Alicia's initiative!). In 1891, the year that Alicia embarked for the United States, she joined the 39 percent of Irish-born people who lived outside Ireland.[50] The population of Ireland decreased at every census between 1841 and 1951, halving its population over that time.[51] Ireland's population has recovered in recent years, but it still remains about a third less than its peak before the famine.

Similar, though less spectacular, versions of the Irish migration unfolded across Europe in the late nineteenth and early twentieth centuries. In the middle of the nineteenth century, millions of Germans migrated, mostly to Pennsylvania and New York. Swedes and Norwegians followed, thousands each year, settling in the upper Midwest of the United States and snapping up cheap (but cold) farmland. After 1890, the drive to migrate shifted southward and eastward to Italy, Spain, Austria-Hungary, and Poland; a new, fast-growing generation of young adults migrated to the United States, Canada, Argentina, and elsewhere. Roughly 55 million, almost all young people, emigrated from Europe between 1850 and 1914.[52]

Migration as the History of Disease

Historians and demographers have studied that European migration, looking for a common explanation for the exodus. Migration in most of these nations was not the result of ecological disaster. It was not restricted to the poorest nations of Europe. As in West Africa today, migrants in nineteenth-century Europe needed resources to finance the journey abroad. Industrialization and the commercialization of agriculture help explain the move to cities, as better agricultural yields released farm hands from the land and higher wages drew them to Birmingham, Cologne, and other factory centers. But emigration from countries like Norway occurred as those nations were just beginning to industrialize. The differences between the wages available in the migrants' home country and those in the destination labor market were an important, but only partial, explanation for the exodus.

Wages in the United States and many European nations started to converge in 1890, and yet migration continued. The presence of friends and family abroad was a draw for the emigrants that followed them, but those network effects played a bigger role in accelerating an emigration once it was well underway.[53]

Changes in demography may provide the best explanation. The economist Richard Easterlin observed that the migration in nineteenth-century Europe occurred more often from countries with surplus young adult populations and high rates of natural increase, usually twenty years after declines in infant mortality.[54] Timothy Hatton and Jeffrey Williamson have expanded on that theory, showing that falling child and infant mortality rates and slower reductions in fertility led to a glut in the labor market for young adults and a disparity in wages with the labor-scarce New World. That created the pressure to emigrate. That pressure was compounded because young adults, who usually struggle the most to find jobs, are also the most willing to emigrate. After the emigration had persisted for some time, the share of young adults in the population declined, wages rose, and the rate of emigration subsided.[55]

Demographic-fueled migration is not just a feature of the nineteenth century. Gordon Hanson and Craig McIntosh have shown that emigration to the United States, Britain, Canada, and Spain was strongly driven by population growth in Latin America, the Middle East, South Asia, and the Caribbean in the 1980s and 1990s.[56] The economist Michael Clemens, a leading expert in migration, has demonstrated that most of the emigration from Mexico to the United States after 1980 can be explained by demographic differences between the two countries. He found that improved child survival in Mexico led to a disproportionate share of young adults and a wage differential with the older, better-paid population living on the US side of the border.[57]

Put in other terms, the history of the decline of infectious diseases has been told through the migration of its beneficiaries. That history began with Western European and Scandinavian nations. As nutrition and incomes improved there at the turn of the nineteenth century, reinforced by greater adoption of breastfeeding, better hygiene, and smallpox vaccination, infant and child mortality rates fell. A decline in fertility in the nations followed, but lagged behind. Twenty years or so later, these additional babies who survived matured into young adults. Those nations that were able to employ some of this disproportionately large number of young adults enjoyed faster economic growth, a demographic dividend. Those who could not be absorbed into the country's workforce were left to migrate.

This pattern can be seen in figure 5.4. It presents the data available on infant mortality and total emigration for the four countries discussed in this chapter. In Mexico, Niger, and Nigeria, the link between the declining rates of infants dying (the dotted lines) and the subsequent accelerating rates of emigration (the solid lines) is apparent, shown here in a distinctive x-pattern. Unfortunately, there is no source of available data on infant mortality in Ireland before 1865. The trend corresponds well, however, with the information known on the improving rates of health and nutrition in predominantly rural Ireland at the turn of the century. Even in 1865, infant mortality remained considerably lower in Ireland than in the more urbanized England and Wales.[58]

Infant Mortality and Total Emigration: Ireland, Mexico, Niger, Nigeria

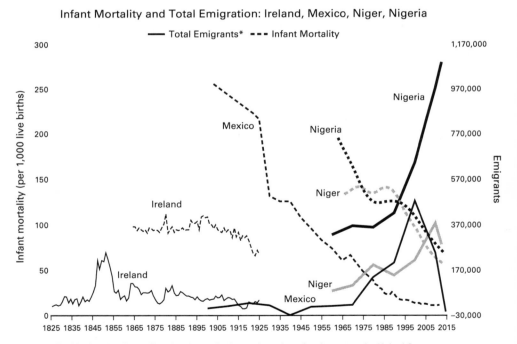

*For Mexico, the data reflect the change in the total number of emigrants to the United States.

Figure 5.4
Data sources: Gapminder, Mexican Migration Project; World Bank, World Development Indicators.

With industrialization and the establishment of sanitation systems, the trends that began in parts of England, Wales, and Scandinavia spread to other Western European nations and eventually to the whole of Europe. After a decade or two, more surviving babies turned into greater numbers of young adults, which led to the beginning of migration from Southern and Eastern Europe around 1890.

Improved health did not arrive in many lower-income nations in East Asia and Latin America until the 1930s or after World War II. It was helped by the invention of antibiotics, the eradication campaigns for malaria and smallpox, and by local governments pioneering new frugal health-care models, like China's barefoot doctors. These changes, again, led to the emergence of a large pool of young adults in those regions. In those East Asian nations where additional men and women were put to work in factories, the economic spoils ensued. But East Asian and Latin American countries that were not able to employ many of these young adults, like the Philippines and Mexico, experienced surges in emigration starting in the late 1960s and 1970s.

Declines of infectious disease and improved childhood survival rates started to take hold in parts of the Middle East and North Africa around the same time as in East Asia and Latin America. But it was not until the immunization campaigns of the Child Survival Revolution, greater use of oral rehydration solution, and more recent efforts to reduce long-neglected diseases did progress in those regions accelerate. In the 1980s and 1990s, those improvements finally reached sub-Saharan Africa and the poorest parts of South Asia too. With child survival improving even in these poorest nations, the current wave of migration from those countries ensued a decade or so later.

These waves of improved infectious disease control fit with regional emigration data, shown in figure 5.5. In each case, more people began moving away from the region roughly fifteen years after the declines in infant and child mortality. The link between infectious disease and migration is not simply a matter of timing. The speed and degree to which the migration occurs also reflects, in part, the way in which those countries managed to reduce those diseases (and the accompanying child mortality rates).

Countries with a slower pace of out-migration following improved health (England in the nineteenth century and Taiwan in the 1960s) are those where the gains in child survival and lower rates of infectious disease have

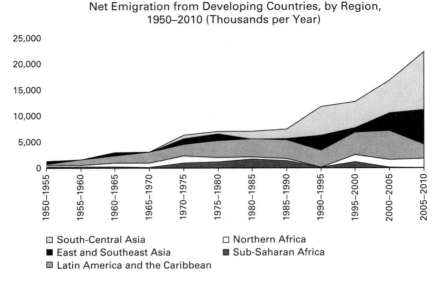

Net Emigration from Developing Countries, by Region,
1950–2010 (Thousands per Year)

□ South-Central Asia   □ Northern Africa
■ East and Southeast Asia   ■ Sub-Saharan Africa
□ Latin America and the Caribbean

Figure 5.5
Data source: UN World Population Prospects.

occurred alongside rising incomes and better job opportunities, improved urban and health infrastructure, and more responsive governance. Nations where the decline in infectious diseases and gains in child survival occurred without these structural changes have experienced faster and more urgent emigration, sometimes at the peril of the migrants. Ireland and Niger are two such examples. Hatton and Williamson theorize that if wage differences between the United States and Europe had been greater or persisted longer, even more emigration might have occurred.[59] In a 2001 paper, these economists also conclude that "exactly the same forces" shaped twentieth-century immigration to Europe and suggest that "there is a good chance that by 2025 Africa will record far greater mass migrations than did nineteenth-century Europe."[60]

These patterns following the decline in infectious diseases may also be seen in the stock of the world's so-called economic migrants. Refugees fleeing war and persecution justifiably garner media attention, but they are small in number in comparison to economic migrants, who move for different reasons, primarily to find better jobs. Between 1965 and 1990, economic migrants remained constant as a share of the world's population, at

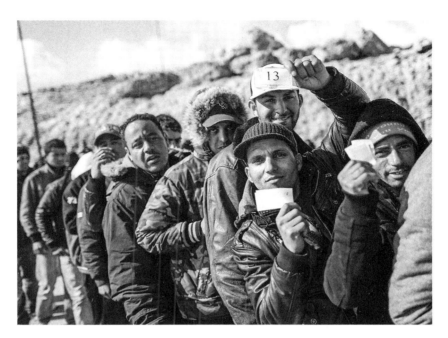

Figure 5.6
Migrants from North and Central Africa waiting in line on the southern island
of Lampedusa, Italy, in 2011. Photo: Reuters/Tony Gentile.

around 2.5 percent, keeping pace with global population growth.[61] With
infant and child mortality improving globally, especially in poorer nations,
the share of economic migrants began to drift slowly upward during the
1990s. By 2000, economic migrants accounted for 2.6 percent of the world's
population. Over the last fifteen years, that migration has accelerated, rising to 3 percent of global population by 2015. Roughly 222 million people
now live outside the countries where they were born, and these migrants
come from different regions of the world than migrants had in the past.[62]

The decline in infectious disease has remade the world through emigration. From the last half of the nineteenth century through the 1930s,
young European migrants to North and South America, Australia, and
South Africa played a major role in the economic development of those
host nations, adding the skills and labor that drove their expanding economies.[63] The United States received two-thirds of this migration and became
the world power that it is today, lifted on the backs of these immigrants. At

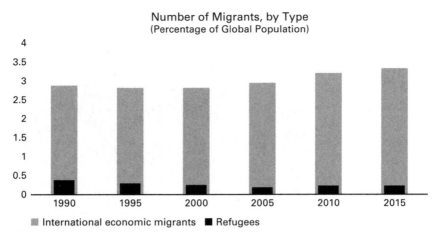

Figure 5.7
Source: World Bank, World Development Indicators.

the same time, that migration benefited the countries they left behind by relieving some of the population pressure and potential social instability in those societies and generating remittances that have at least helped reduce poverty, if not expand those economies.[64]

The World Is Getting Better in Worrisome Ways

Migration is frequently viewed as the product of desperate circumstances. People are pushed from their homes and pulled to the relative safety and prosperity offered elsewhere. But economic migration is more properly viewed as the by-product of success, twenty years or so removed. It arises as populations free themselves from the plagues, parasites, and early death that have characterized human existence for millennia. The volume and pace of the migration that ensues reflects how ready those nations are to accommodate the aspirations and basic needs of their growing number of young adults.

Many nations are not ready. In recent decades, it has become possible to reduce the burden of infectious diseases in poor nations with medical invention, the generosity and initiatives of international donors, and the hard work and frugal innovations of local governments. Fewer children being doomed to die unnecessarily simply because of the geography of their birth is a tremendous achievement. The rate at which infant and child mortality occurs should become rarer still. But celebrating that success should not mean ignoring the challenges that will arise in nations that have not yet built the health-care systems needed to care for these soon-to-be adults, the urban infrastructure to house them, or the robust, labor-intensive economies to employ them.

The World Bank estimates that the working-age population (more than 15 years old) in developing countries will increase by 2.1 billion by 2050. If national employment stays at the rate in 2015, only 1.2 billion of those people will find jobs in their own country, leaving the remaining nearly 900 million in search of work. Of that population, 333 million will come from sub-Saharan Africa, 283 million from South Asia, and 120 million will be from the Middle East and North Africa.[65]

To date, climate change and extreme weather have played only minor roles in overall international migration. The International Displacement Monitoring Center estimates that 19 million people were displaced by natural disasters in 2015.[66] But most of the migration that resulted has been internal, occurring within the same country. With rising sea levels, more drought and desertification, and higher rates of crop failures, that pattern may change and lead to even greater numbers of people leaving their countries and moving abroad.[67]

Ultimately, it is the job of those young adults, local activists, and their national governments to undertake the long, hard struggle of advancing the political and social reforms needed to adapt to demographic change and the partial success of declining rates of infectious diseases. But donors and international institutions should recognize that lower-income nations are confronting these large-scale changes at a faster rate and with fewer resources than in the past. International initiatives have not focused on supporting nations in their efforts to reduce congestion in health and urban infrastructure or to address noncommunicable diseases and the employment needs of adults. The final chapter of this book outlines a few ideas on how these nations and social reformers might be better supported in their efforts.

But there should also be greater recognition that the transition that is now unfolding in lower-income nations was not always pretty in wealthier nations and that it has always been accompanied by migration. The difference is that the mass emigration from nineteenth-century Europe had the good fortune of occurring at a time when the international environment for migration was largely unrestrained. At that time, migration was even encouraged, by both the sending and receiving nations.[68] In the aftermath of World War II, many Western European nations reactivated their migration promotion schemes with traditional receiving countries, such as Australia, New Zealand, and Canada.[69] Refugees from Eastern and Central Europe, including my parents, who fled revolution and the ashes of war from behind the Iron Curtain, were welcomed, for the most part, in the United States and other Western nations.[70] This situation continued through the 1960s, but it no longer exists for lower-income nations and their young adults today.

With the oil crisis in the early 1970s and the decline in economic fortunes of Western nations, governments began to make greater efforts to restrict immigration and the movement of refugees and undocumented workers. In 1976, a poll that the United Nations Secretariat conducted of its member states found only ten nations that indicated immigration rates were "too high." A 2011 poll found that number had more than tripled, to thirty-three countries.[71] That shift in views has been reflected in the adoption of stricter immigration policies. More emphasis is now put on the skills and resources of migrants, with many nations moving to "points"-based visas, skilled employment-based work visas, temporary business visas, student visas, and investor visas.[72] In early 2018, US president Donald Trump urged a Congressional delegation to adopt a version of that system, using blunt and reportedly vulgar language to call for more migrants from developed countries, citing Norway in particular, and fewer from impoverished Haiti and African nations.[73]

Undoubtedly, the race and religion of the current pool of migrants has played a role in such sentiments. For example, there is a clear need for low-cost labor to assist the growing number of elderly in Western nations. With the baby boomer generation aging and fertility rates declining, the number of people over 65 is soaring in rich countries. In the United States, that population is expected to reach 72 million in 2030. The number of centenarians in wealthy nations is doubling every decade and is expected to approach four million by 2050.[74] There are millions of capable and underemployed people who could immigrate to Europe, Japan, or America to care for the elderly and infirm, provide them emotional support, and monitor their medication. And, yet, substantial investments are being made in the research and development of robots to provide elder care instead.[75] I asked Tyler Cowen, who has studied the role of automation in the global economy, to explain these investments given the large pool of available immigrant labor and the potential human contact they might provide. He replied: "Voters will prefer robots."[76]

Recent history affirms Cowen's intuition. In high-income countries, politicians who have not responded to the concerns of the public over assimilating migrants with different races, religions, and unfamiliar cultural and social customs have failed to do so at their peril. The results of the UK's referendum on withdrawing from the European Union and the 2016 presidential race in the United States surprised many observers, but they reflected the public's great and growing unease with immigration.

It is unclear how much the restrictions and increasingly hostile attitudes toward immigration have managed to deter migration. The arrival of legal immigrants has likely been reduced, but restrictive policies and measures may have also had the unintended consequence of encouraging irregular and illegal immigration, delaying assimilation, and spurring the permanent settlement of migrant workers who can no longer travel back and forth to their home nations. It is possible that more thoughtful, redoubled efforts to reduce immigration may have a greater effect in the future. Yet, that effort puts many Western nations in the perverse situation of working hard to restrict the movement of migrants who are, in part, the natural result of the progress in health that those same Western nations helped fund.

In sum, the world has gotten better in ways that should make us worry. The last two decades have brought dramatic reductions in endemic infectious disease and child mortality, but not the improvements in health-care systems, responsive governance, and employment opportunities that accompanied these changes in wealthier nations in the past. Rapid population growth, unprecedented urbanization, and an increase in the share of young adults are straining the capacity of governments and ecosystems while spurring migration, instability, and the risk of pandemic diseases and chronic ailments. These challenges are amplified both by the sluggishness of many donors to adapt to the perils of partial success and by the more restrictive trade and immigration policies of many developed governments. It is not hard to envision that the next two decades in lower-income nations may be more violent and conflict-filled than the last, reversing some of the great progress that has recently occurred.

We should worry, but, more importantly, we should act. The next chapter proposes recommendations for how the global community—international institutions, foreign aid agencies, philanthropists, policymakers, and the readers of this book—can assist lower-income nations to confront the paradoxical progress made in our long fight against infectious diseases.

6 The Exoneration of William H. Stewart

The time has come to close the book on infectious diseases. We have basically wiped out infection in the United States.
—Attributed to William H. Stewart, US Surgeon General, 1967 or 1968

William H. Stewart accomplished a great deal as Surgeon General at a consequential moment in the history of US public health. Stewart, a pediatrician and epidemiologist, held the post of "America's doctor" when it carried considerably more power than it does now and was responsible for the day-to-day administration of the US Public Health Service.[1] He was appointed in 1965, one year after his predecessor, Luther Terry, had issued a bombshell report linking cigarette smoking to higher rates of lung cancer and other diseases. Stewart managed to get the first health warning labels on cigarette packs, which required facing down the US tobacco industry at the height of its influence and at a time when 42 percent of American adults smoked.[2] The year 1965 was also when Lyndon Johnson enacted Medicare and Medicaid, which provided health insurance to older and disabled Americans, and one year after the landmark Civil Rights Act. Stewart threatened to withhold federal funds from hospitals that refused to integrate their staff and open their doors to minority patients. He also drew the link between air pollution and lung disease, which helped set the stage for the enactment of the Clean Air Act of 1970. Stewart raged against the "glass curtain" that separated the poor from quality care, built health facilities in underserved areas, and launched a campaign to vaccinate more than 100 million people in Africa against smallpox and measles.[3]

But for all his accomplishments, Stewart might be best known now for claiming that the United States had overcome the threat of infectious disease and it was time to move on. That quote surfaced in the early days of the HIV epidemic and has been used in dozens of books, reports, and articles that warn of the perils of complacency on emerging infectious diseases and antibiotic resistance. For the medical community, Stewart's quote has become the equivalent of the advertisements for the "unsinkable" *Titanic*—an apt metaphor for humanity's hubris in grappling with microbes that can never truly be defeated. Stewart died in 2008 and the obituaries for him that appeared in the *New York Times* and the prestigious British medical journal the *Lancet* both cited the statement.[4]

Stewart's line about turning the page on infectious disease has become, according to the *New Yorker* magazine, "one of modern medicine's more famous quotes."[5] The only problem is that Stewart never said it.

Brad Spellberg and Bonnie Taylor-Blake, physicians and medical researchers, spent years looking for the provenance of the Stewart quote. They worked with the historian for the US Public Health Service and searched every conceivable archive and database. Spellberg and Taylor-Blake traced the quote to a 1989 US National Institute of Allergy and Infectious Diseases (NIAID) meeting on emerging viruses. The HIV epidemic raged unabated at that time and one of the speakers condemned US complacency in preparing for such pandemics. In doing so, he cited Stewart as an example of that complacency, referencing a purported statement that Stewart had made at a 1968 conference claiming that science had probed the frontiers of knowledge about infectious diseases. As it turns out, the speaker had not attended the conference at which Stewart spoke. Several journalists were present at the NIAID meeting and in their subsequent reporting, the reference to Stewart evolved into a direct quote, with some citing Stewart's 1968 speech and others noting an earlier one in 1967. And so, an urban legend was born. Spellberg and Taylor-Blake write that the "spectacularly erroneous quote has been cited innumerable times to underscore ongoing public health problems caused by antibiotic-resistant and emerging infections."[6] Michael Specter, a well-known science writer, did not originate the quote, but penned an apology to Stewart for having used it in several pieces over the years.[7]

The story of the misquoting of William Stewart is not included in this book to embarrass those who have mistakenly cited the quote over the years. We all work hard to avoid mistakes, but some happen regardless. Indeed, despite my best efforts, there are undoubtedly some even in this book.

Moreover, while those who cited the Stewart quote were wrong, their underlying point is not. In the 1950s and 1960s, there were leading US

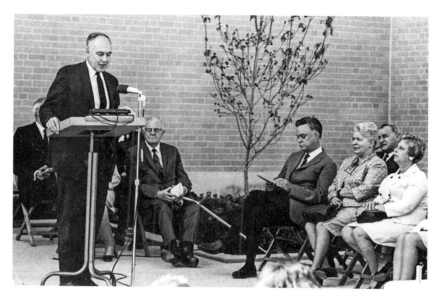

Figure 6.1

William H. Stewart speaks at Johns Hopkins University School of Hygiene and Public Health on September 18, 1968. Photo: William C. Hamilton, Courtesy of the Alan Mason Chesney Medical Archives of the Johns Hopkins Medical Institutions.

medical researchers other than Stewart who were skeptical of the continued relevance of infectious disease.[8] The United States was (and remains) woefully ill-prepared for the threat of antibiotic resistance and future pandemics.

But the Stewart episode is also noteworthy for what he did say in those speeches, not only for what he did not. In that 1967 speech to the Sixty-fifth Annual Meeting of the Association of State and Territorial Health Officers, Stewart emphasized that the "warning flags are still flying in the communicable disease field. ... While we are engaged in taking on new duties ... we cannot and must not lose sight of our traditional program responsibilities."[9] Rather than arguing for moving beyond infectious disease, Stewart emphasized the need for continued vigilance against the threat of plagues and parasites even amid changing health needs. That need continues today, and this book should not be taken to suggest otherwise.

The risk of dangerous disease events is ever-present, with the continued emergence of new plagues, such as HIV/AIDS, and the evolution of existing microbes, especially influenza. The risk of such emerging infectious diseases

may be greater than ever with warming temperatures, increased urbanization, the industrialization of agriculture, and higher volumes of trade and
travel. Some cancers, such as cervical cancer, are often caused by infectious
disease, and many believe there is a link between infection and diabetes.
The US Centers for Disease Control and Prevention reported that more than
two million people in the United States are infected with antibiotic-resistant
bacteria annually, and 23,000 die as a result.[10] An estimated 200,000 people
die each year from multidrug-resistant tuberculosis worldwide. Continued
global progress against infectious diseases is not inevitable and, without our
attention and sustained investment, it could easily be reversed.

But the need for continued vigilance against microbes should not obscure
the dramatic progress made in controlling the everyday toll of infectious diseases, nor should it keep us from adapting to the changes brought on by that
progress. This is the point that Stewart made in his 1968 speech at Johns
Hopkins University, and it is worth quoting at length. Stewart said:

> Powerful tools have been developed to characterize these diseases in man and in
> society—the tools of microbiology, epidemiology, and biostatistics…means for
> preventing or alleviating disease in an individual or en masse have been devel-
> oped and applied…and never before in man's history has a society reached such
> a peak of health.
>
> This success story brings us to the here and now. And largely as a result of this
> success story, times have changed. The purpose of our efforts—the preservation
> and improvement of health—can no longer be measured on the scale of microbi-
> ology. Our exploitation of that science has just about caught up with the frontiers
> of public need. Clearly we cannot turn our backs on microbiology—certain nota-
> ble gaps remain in our knowledge and capability, and maintenance of a vigilant
> effort will always be required.
>
> But just as clearly the characterization of health in terms of microbiology and
> infectious disease epidemiology cannot serve as the base for our future endeavors.
> Rather, the moving tides of society, which we have helped to move, are compelling
> us to redefine our purposes in quite different terms—the terms of man's adaptation
> to his total environment.
>
> Immediately we find ourselves on dark and shaky ground. This new definition
> of purpose rests on sciences much less comfortably exact than microbiology. We
> find the familiar equations of one cause-one disease disappearing into a complex
> of multiple causation.[11]

This is a fairly accurate characterization of the US public health situation in
1968, the progress that had occurred, and the challenges that lay ahead. As
figure 6.2 shows, infectious disease-related deaths in the United States had

declined precipitously in the prior decades (with the significant exception of the 1918 flu epidemic). US deaths from infectious diseases rose again with the HIV epidemic in the first half of the 1990s, but reached nowhere near historical levels. Mortality rates from infectious diseases have fallen since 1995 and reached unprecedented lows in the past two decades. The progress against the noninfectious disease threats that Stewart worried about, such as smoking or pollution, has not been nearly as sharp. So while the threat that pandemic disease and antibiotic resistance pose to the United States continues to loom large, Stewart was right that infectious disease epidemiology should no longer be the exclusive frame through which the United States views its health. During Stewart's tenure, the US Public Health Service launched a major national vaccination campaign against measles, but it also created a system of regional medical centers to tackle stroke, heart disease, and cancer, the diseases that had emerged as the leading killers of Americans.[12]

In recent decades, the same progress that Stewart observed in the United States in controlling plagues and parasites has begun to extend worldwide, even into the poorest regions of the world. Infectious diseases now cause less than one-fifth of the total death and disability in South Asia and less than 44 percent in sub-Saharan Africa. The health transition occurring in many

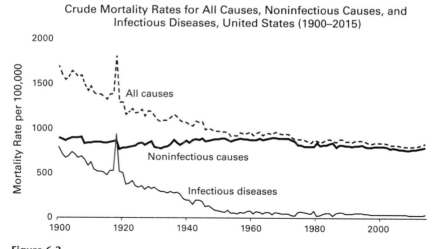

Figure 6.2

Data sources: Armstrong, Conn, and Pinner, "Trends in Infectious Disease Mortality," 1999; Institute for Health Metrics and Evaluation, GBD 2015.

poor nations is much faster than in the past. In 2040, Bangladesh, a country that the World Bank defines as low-income, will have roughly the same share of its health burden dominated by cancer, heart diseases, and other noncommunicable diseases as the United States does today. The difference is that in the United States, that transition occurred over more than a hundred years. In Bangladesh, it will have happened in a third of the time and at a much lower level of income. The health-care systems in many developing nations are completely unprepared for this rapid change. Without access to government-provided chronic and preventative care or the personal wealth to buy it, young, working-age people in poor countries are experiencing staggering increases in noncommunicable illnesses. Four of those diseases—cancer, upper respiratory illnesses, heart disease, and diabetes—already account for nearly six of ten of global deaths annually, yet only 1 percent of development assistance for health is dedicated to noncommunicable diseases.

The speech that Stewart made in 1968 argued for broadening the US approach to health concerns and grappling with the consequences—for good and ill—that had come with the progress made in controlling infectious disease. That argument applies with equal force to many poorer nations now. Dr. Agnes Binagwaho, the former permanent secretary of the Rwandan Ministry of Health, has said: "noncommuncIable diseases are often considered the problem of middle- and high-income countries. ... I want to stand strongly against that."[13]

The rise in these chronic diseases is only one example of the ways that the decline in infectious diseases has, to paraphrase Stewart, moved the tides of society in poorer nations, a move that global health initiatives helped bring about. The implications of that shift extend beyond health, and many of those consequences are profoundly positive. Reductions in infectious diseases have helped raise new economic empires, shift the geography and character of human settlement, and spur the grand movements of people toward a better life. But some of the changes are more worrisome. The growth of many poor world cities is far outpacing their infrastructure, leaving nearly a billion people living in slums. Lack of sufficient jobs for young adults is breeding instability and spurring desperate attempts at migration. Climate change and increased hostility to trade and immigration in the United States and Europe are raising the temperature on a stew of demographic changes that already seems poised to boil over. It is not hard to envision a scenario where the next two decades are even less peaceful than the last.

In short, the history of the decline in infectious diseases has been at least as consequential as the story of their rise. But grappling with the consequences of the partial progress against infectious disease in poorer nations is, as Stewart put it, "dark and shaky ground" that requires confronting "a complex of multiple causation."

Confronting the Complex of Multiple Causation

Developing countries face multiple challenges: retooling their health-care systems to provide cost-effective preventive and chronic care; improving the reach and sustainability of urban infrastructure; attracting private investment and increasing formal employment opportunities; and extending the progress against infectious diseases, extreme poverty, and undernutrition to those who still suffer from these conditions. High-income countries, including the United States, share these problems, too. The difference is that demographic changes are forcing poorer nations to confront them faster, with fewer resources, amid a changing climate and a more hostile geopolitical environment for trade and immigration.

It is easy to be pessimistic about the prospects for those lower-income countries facing these challenges. But we should not lose sight of the fact that the decline of infectious diseases presents an historic opportunity to invest in the large young adult populations flooding the rapidly growing cities of developing nations as the best hope for generating more inclusive economic prosperity. Cities can be more productive and healthful than rural settings. Urban productivity and healthfulness, if not overwhelmed by traffic and clogged infrastructure, improves with population size and better education.[14] Solutions to these challenges will necessarily be context-specific, but here are three broad areas that developing country governments should consider investing in when facing the paradox of progress against infectious diseases.

First, there is no quick or ready-made fix for creating sustainable urban infrastructure in sprawling poor world cities, but instituting the right incentives can help. Many residents of developing-country cities, especially those living in slums, lack clear property titles to their homes. Establishing easy-to-enforce land rights can promote investment in formal housing, free workers to move to find jobs and get access to city services, and establish the foundation for a property tax system. With the resulting resources and a bit of empowerment from national governments, city governments may be freer to do more to improve their business environments, ease bureaucratic constraints on small- and medium-sized enterprises, and attract private infrastructure investment. Municipal governments may also prove more capable than national authorities in responding to the demographic pressures and environmental challenges that poor world cities face.[15] A World Bank study of African cities providing the best water services to the poor found mayors behind several of the success stories, including those of Durban, South Africa and Nyeri, Kenya.[16]

Second, cities, health-care systems, and economies succeed when their participants have the knowledge and communication skills to pursue and spread new ideas.[17] This requires a good education. Despite dramatic increases in school attendance, many lower-income nations continue to lag far behind their wealthy country counterparts in capabilities such as reading fluently, solving practical problems with arithmetic, and critical reasoning.[18]

Lower-income nations, especially in sub-Saharan Africa, are in dire need of more investment in human capital. With declines in infectious diseases and steeply rising rates of child survival, more sub-Saharan Africans will reach the ages of prime employment (ages 15 to 64) by 2035 than will be added by the rest of the world combined.[19] While sub-Saharan Africa has greatly increased school attendance, it is still the worst-performing region in educational outcomes. Up to 40 percent of children in the region do not meet basic learning outcomes in numeracy, and half fall short in literacy.[20] In 2016, Ellen Johnson Sirleaf, the president of Liberia, took a radical step to address the problem of failing schools, absentee teachers, and missing books: she delegated management of ninety-three public elementary schools to eight different private contractors. Despite higher costs and more variation in performance across the contractors, the results after one year showed, on average, a 60 percent improvement in educational outcomes in the privately run schools.[21] More assessment of the Liberian experiment is needed, but the early results are promising.[22] Private providers of public education are certainly not the solution everywhere, but they may help improve school attendance and quality in nations with high rates of corruption and poor public services. If so, it will be important to continue to monitor performance and guard against the inequitable access that may arise with privately run schools.[23]

Third, a strong primary health-care system can be a cost-effective way to manage many ills, from enabling early identification of a new disease outbreak to finding a young woman's breast cancer before her tumor is ulcerated and past the stage where it can be treated. But many developing countries have shown too little interest in primary health care. Poorer nations have tended to invest in expensive hospitals that cater to the needs of local elites.[24] For example, the *Economist* recently reported that the number of primary-care providers in China declined 6 percent between 2002 and 2013, while hospital capacity almost doubled. The number of hospital beds per person in China now exceeds that in the United States.[25]

High-quality primary care is not beyond the means of many developing countries; those countries that have instituted it have achieved dramatic health improvements. Brazil's family health program covers more than half of the population, costs the government roughly $50 per person, and has sharply reduced the number of deaths from heart disease, diabetes, and infectious diseases.[26] Community health worker programs that use low-cost, simple diagnostics and digital technologies can extend basic health care to the poor in rural areas and slums.[27] Developing countries that have invested in their own capacity to generate and apply evidence-based, localized health policies, like Mexico, have made the greatest gains in public health.[28]

The Role of Aid in Adapting to the Decline of Infectious Diseases

Determining a country's priorities and allocating scarce resources in the face of its demographic challenges are ultimately the responsibility of national governments and local civil society, which have the most at stake in the future of their own nation. Aid represents a small and diminishing share of overall investment to lower-income countries. Moreover, aid agencies and other donors are also outsiders, poorly positioned to undertake the sustained, hard struggle of adapting institutional and social reforms to local needs and advancing them on behalf of lower-income countries.

Past foreign aid initiatives succeeded in delivering food, cash, drugs, and other technologies to the world's poor, even in countries with dysfunctional governments. But donors and international agencies have a dismal record of advancing the political and social reforms that would help poorer nations seize the potential of their improved health. Donors cannot manage primary health-care systems in other countries or enforce sensible regulations on tobacco, land use, or air pollution. Aid agencies and philanthropists have had little success creating economic growth and employment in other nations, let alone installing democratic and responsive governance or sustainable urban planning. It is hard for bilateral donors, reliant on the opinions of their domestic constituents, to justify investments in infrastructure that local governments are ultimately responsible for providing: roads, bridges, sewers, and hospitals. It is the height of hubris to believe that philanthropy and foreign aid can stop the social, political, and economic forces that lead young adults to aspire to a better life and emigrate.

But that doesn't mean foreign aid officials, philanthropists, policymakers, and other readers of this book cannot assist lower-income nations in their difficult tasks. Progress will depend on mobilizing more support for changing the way international assistance seeks to advance health and development in poorer nations.

In Stewart's 1968 speech, he spoke of the need for humankind to adapt to the changes in the total environment, brought on in part by the decline in infectious diseases. Below are three critical points that should serve as benchmarks for assessing international initiatives and their engagement on that agenda.

First, if international development initiatives are going to remain effective as a means of advancing health and economic development, they must be more responsive to the changing needs of lower-income nations. This may sound like an obvious point. But it requires making existing aid and health programs less focused on donor-directed inputs—specific disease-reduction targets, years of primary schooling, and "dollar a day" poverty—and more concerned with local outcomes such as learning, capable economies and governments, and better health, especially among the poor and disenfranchised. At a 2013 conference dedicated to ending child mortality globally, Richard Cash, the co-inventor of the oral rehydration solution that saved so many lives, now a professor at the Harvard School of Public Health, said:

> By simply focusing on mortality, which so much of the focus has been on, we ignore issues such as contaminated water, such as poor educational systems … that other package of development issues which are critical. What we don't want is successes in mortality and people still living in abject poverty, and in fact that is what has happened. Our tools are very powerful, our vaccines are very good, our interventions are really good, but we haven't adequately addressed the underlying risks and causes of both the mortality and the morbidity.[29]

Global health priorities must also include the noncommunicable diseases and associated health risks that now cause the largest proportion of premature death and disability in lower-income nations. It is simply not sustainable to commit substantial resources to fighting one set of treatable and preventable diseases only to watch the very same patients die prematurely as a result of equally treatable and preventable conditions. The 2017 launch of Resolve to Save Lives, a $225 million initiative that seeks to improve hypertension control in lower-income countries, provides hope for more donor interest in the rising tide of noncommunicable disease.[30] The extensive platforms that the US government and other donors have built to combat HIV/AIDS and other infectious diseases also provide a positive legacy. For example, most international infectious disease initiatives have facilities to ensure the provision of affordable, quality-assured medicines; allowing lower-income countries to use those facilities to procure essential drugs for cancer, diabetes, or noncommunicable diseases would require the assent of donors like the United States, the United Kingdom, and the Bill and Melinda Gates Foundation. Providing that support for expanding those global programs that provide lifesaving commodities and services will be important, particularly for the poorest slums and most conflict-ridden states that face a crippling dual challenge of infectious and noncommunicable diseases.

The United States and other donors should recast their global health aid programs from disease-focused goals to more outcome-oriented measures for improving health in the targeted countries and populations. Adopting a patient-centered approach based on health outcomes rather than disease-specific reduction targets, and investing in data collection to monitor it, would increase the accountability and capability of global health investments. That would make those global health programs more valuable and easier for governments of lower-income nations to move from being largely dependent on outside aid to operating the health programs themselves. Ensuring that developing countries have greater say in choosing the outcome measures chosen will improve their utility and increase the likelihood of their eventual local adoption.

Central to understanding how to advance the interests of those in need is listening to what they actually want. In 2015, Angus Deaton and Robert Tortora analyzed data from multiple polls averaged across sub-Saharan Africa and found that respondents prioritize a better livelihood—new jobs and agricultural improvements—over gains in health care. This does not mean aid initiatives should no longer prioritize health, where they have been most effective. Evidence suggests respondents' desire for additional health aid may have declined in part because infectious disease has lessened and their greater satisfaction with the existing aid programs.[31] It does suggest, however, the need to pair future health aid with more investment in other areas that may also help firms and factories, large and small, employ people productively.

Education is another example of where an outcome-based approach may help. Lant Pritchett, in his book *The Rebirth of Education*, argues that the dogged pursuit of the global goal of universal primary school attendance has obscured the lack of achievement in the underlying objective of education: learning. The United Nations Sustainable Development Goals, released in 2015, include objectives on educational quality, but there is no agreement on how to measure progress. Many countries resist being compared to their peers and there are often wide discrepancies between official literacy rates and those reported in surveys.[32] In 2017, the World Bank announced an initiative that may help. It will compile a Human Capital Project, an annual evidence-based and transparent assessment that will combine measures of health outcomes and educational quality along with a country's gross domestic productivity. The idea is to encourage private sector firms to use this index in their foreign investment decisions, thereby creating a strong financial incentive for governments to devote more resources to better education and health.

Thoughtful and targeted investments can also help lower-income nations confront the demographic challenges that come with the decline in infectious diseases. In recent years, donors have increased investments in voluntary family planning and girls' education. These programs have helped to reduce fertility in nations like Senegal to more sustainable levels and better integrate women into the economy. These investments should be increased. Recent efforts to encourage private investors to put their money toward building infrastructure and electricity generation, such as the Obama administration's Power Africa initiative, can make it easier for factories and entrepreneurs to open businesses and hire more young workers.

The second step on the road to a less worrisome future is for philanthropists and foreign aid agencies to embrace a more limited but still useful role in helping poor and emerging economies confront the demographic challenges that have accompanied declining rates of infectious disease. This role should focus on funding the data collection and research that advocates and activists need to advance locally inspired change. This effort should include providing the resources and technical support that local researchers and governments need to test their best ideas and working with those local actors to reduce the results to implementable, evidence-based programs. Outsiders can, where appropriate, also provide a useful service by supporting social reformers in pressing their governments for the adoption of the better policies and by monitoring, evaluating, and publishing the results to hold local governments and donors accountable.

Bloomberg Philanthropies, a philanthropic institution that supports some of my research, has used this strategy to help poor and emerging economies advance tobacco control.[33] In 2008, for example, Turkey raised cigarette taxes to account for 81 percent of the total price of a pack and banned tobacco advertising and smoking in public places. The next year, admissions for smoking-related disease to hospital emergency rooms in Turkey fell by nearly a quarter; smoking rates declined 16 percent over three years.[34] The Philippines has also recently adopted similar reforms.[35] This data-supported, locally driven strategy on tobacco control has worked in poor and wealthy countries alike and in the face of fierce opposition from the multibillion-dollar cigarette industry. There is no reason it cannot be used to help advance reform on other issues: more capable health-care systems, family planning, and higher-quality education for girls.

Third, politicians in the United States, Europe, and other wealthy nations must come to terms with the inconsistencies in their policies on climate change, global health, trade, and immigration. Failure to face the reality of climate change and its causes is hurting the economies of many lower-income countries, threatens to undermine progress on global health, and may accelerate the rates of international migration. Researchers have identified, for example, a link between the effects of climate change (declining rainfall and warming temperatures) and childhood stunting in Kenya since 1975.[36] Many of the fast-expanding cities in lower-income countries are on the coast or downstream from great rivers. This puts Guayaquil, Ecuador; Ho Chi Minh City, Vietnam; and Khulna, Bangladesh, for example, among the cities that are most vulnerable to floods caused by global warming.[37]

Politicians in the United States and Europe are increasingly campaigning for office—and sometimes winning—on a policy of anti-immigration and economic nationalism. A mandate from voters should be respected, but wiser politicians and policymakers, rather than exploit the fears of their constituents, would also recognize and explain to voters that those policies work at cross-purposes. Protectionism undermines economic growth and job creation in emerging economies. In the near term, rising incomes and employment opportunities alone will not stop immigrants from countries with recent declines in infectious disease, but they may shorten the duration and intensity of that migration. Voters in Europe and the United States can choose to be antitrade or anti-immigration, but it is hard to achieve both goals at the same time.

In a globalizing world, little stays local for long. Increasingly, what happens within the borders of any country can affect many others. This is certainly true for the demographic challenges spurred by the partial success in controlling infectious disease. Richard Haass, the president of the Council on Foreign Relations, has called for greater adoption of the notion of sovereign obligation, in which governments have obligations to control the risks and policies in their territory that could adversely affect others.[38] It is a doctrine of hard-nosed self-interest and necessity, and an idea that applies with equal force in this context. Lower-income nations must move quickly to adapt to their demographic changes and seize the opportunities offered by their improving health. But wealthy governments must also recognize their obligation to do no harm to those efforts with shortsighted positions on climate change and overly restrictive policies on trade and immigration. One of the best ways to assist poorer nations is to stop obstructing them from undertaking appropriate measures to help themselves. The notion of sovereign obligation is a recipe for intergovernmental cooperation in a world where the day-to-day threat of infectious diseases is diminishing. It is an idea that, together with the other recommendations advocated here, could help make the world not only better, but also less worrisome.

The Myth of the Good Epidemic

The historian Christopher Hamlin has cautioned against the "myth of the good epidemic," the notion that new outbreaks of cholera, tuberculosis, and other infectious scourges might motivate needed investment in sanitation and other positive government reforms, as some argue occurred in the past.[39] I also do not subscribe to that myth. The lessons of the past are not that controlling infectious disease and improving the health of the poorest are too much trouble or that progress against pestilence came prematurely to developing nations. There is no worthier goal than reducing unnecessary pain and early death, especially among children.

At the same time, many governments and nonprofits working to promote better health in poorer nations fail to consider that declining mortality rates from infectious disease—the goal that many count as their primary index of progress—will also bring profound challenges if not paired with broader gains in economic development, governance, education, and infrastructure. It is only through an improved understanding of the difficulties in the path that has been taken to reduce infectious diseases that these future obstacles can be overcome, forewarned with a more realistic sense of the deep challenges that lie ahead.

Acknowledgments

Writing a book is like swimming across an ocean: no one can do it for you, but you would be foolish to attempt the long journey without the support of people you trust. I am indebted to the friends, family, and colleagues who kept me from losing my way over the course of this project. Binya Appelbaum, Steve Davis, Joe Dieleman, Trish Dorff, David Fidler, Betsy Fuller, Eric Goosby, Richard Haass, Kelly Henning, Olivia Judson, Ruth Levine, Jim Lindsay, Chris Murray, Devi Sridhar, and Gina Suh all read drafts of this book and offered invaluable advice and criticism. Also helpful were the incisive comments provided by Alyssa Ayres, John Campbell, and Michael Clemens on particular chapters. I am likewise grateful to David Bishai, Mushtaque Chowdhury, Tyler Cowen, Chris Dye, Alez Ezeh, Ed Glaeser, Miriam Gross, Mark Harrison, David Nalin, Ole Norheim, Steve Radelet, and Dean Spears for their suggestions and insights. Sabine Baumgartner, Daniel Burke, Kaitlin Christenson, and Monique Libby generously located exhibits that appear in this book. Lisa Ortiz and Amanda Shendruk gave great advice that immeasurably improved the design and clarity of the figures and maps in this book. My thanks also to the anonymous reviewers of the manuscript for their unsparing and constructive critiques. Any errors that remain in this book are mine, as are all the views expressed.

Throughout this project I was fortunate to have tremendous research assistance, most especially from Matthew Cohen, who assisted in the data collection, analysis, fact checking, and editing of this text. I am also grateful to Caroline Andridge who was my research assistant when this book was conceived. My thanks also to Tara Templin, who was a consultant on research related to this book, and to all the interns who toiled on improving the manuscript: Jude Alawa, Birdy Assefa, Merykokeb Belay, Kofi Gunu, Ewodaghe Harrell, Stephanie McKay, and Yuqian Zhang.

I am indebted to Bloomberg Philanthropies for financial support for research incorporated into this book. I am also grateful to the Rockefeller Foundation, which granted me a writing residency at the beautiful Villa Serbelloni, Bellagio, where I conceived the broad outline of this book. Julia Fromholz did a heroic edit of an early draft of this book, sending her hand-written comments from Islamabad, page by page, via an iPhone camera. Tom Redburn edited this manuscript twice and vastly improved the text with his sharp eye and terrific blend of constructive criticism and warm encouragement. Finally, my thanks to my literary agent Andrew Wylie, and Bob Prior, Judy Feldmann, and Anne-Marie Bono at the MIT Press, for their enthusiastic support and enduring contributions to this book.

Every writer of a book thanks family, but truly this book would never have happened without the love and support of mine. Paul Bollyky was a sounding board throughout the production of this book and knew I could write it even when I did not. Andrea Bollyky Purcell and Laszlo Bollyky read drafts of the manuscript, endured my endless complaints, and provided constant encouragement. My greatest appreciation goes to my wife, Brooke, who did without me for far too long because of this book, but never stopped believing in it, or in me.

Notes

Preface

1. *Historical Statistics of the United States*, millennial edition online, ed. Susan B. Carter, Scott Sigmund Gartner, Michael R. Haines, Alan L. Olmstead, Richard Sutch, and Gavin Wright (Cambridge: Cambridge University Press, 2006), tables Ab912–927, http://hsus.cambridge.org/HSUSWeb/HSUSEntryServlet.

2. Angus Maddison, *Contours of the World Economy 1–2030 AD* (Oxford: Oxford University Press, 2007), table 3; World Bank Group, "New Country Classifications by Income Level: 2017–2018," World Bank blog, July 1, 2017, https://blogs.worldbank .org/opendata/new-country-classifications-income-level-2017-2018.

3. *Historical Statistics of the United States*, tables Vc793–797; Samuel Preston and Michael R. Haines, *Fatal Years* (Princeton, NJ: Princeton University Press, 1996), 51, 198–199, 208; Robert William Fogel, *The Escape from Hunger and Premature Death, 1700–2100: Europe, America, and the Third World* (Cambridge: Cambridge University Press, 2004), 2; Clayne L. Pope, "Adult Mortality in America before 1900: A View from Family Histories," in *Strategic Factors in Nineteenth Century American Growth: A Volume to Honor Robert W. Fogel*, ed. Claudia Goldin and Hugh Rockoff (Chicago: University of Chicago Press for NBER, 1992), 267–296.

4. Douglas C. Ewbank and Samuel H. Preston, "Personal Health Behaviour and the Decline in Infant and Child Mortality in the United States 1900–1930," in *What We Know about the Health Transition: The Cultural Social and Behavioural Determinants of Health*, ed. John Caldwell et al. (Canberra: Australian National University, 1990), 116–149; Preston and Haines, *Fatal Years*, 4–6; Stanford T. Shulman, "The History of Pediatric Infectious Disease," *Pediatric Research* 55 (2004): 163–176.

5. Nancy Schrom Dye and Daniel Blake Smith, "Mother Love and Infant Death, 1750–1920," *Journal of American History* 73 (1986): 329–353.

6. Hans Zinsser, *Rats, Lice and History* (New York: Black Dog & Leventhal, 1935), 13.

7. Robert J. Gordon, *The Rise and Fall of American Growth* (Princeton, NJ: Princeton University Press, 2016), 209.

8. The drop in life expectancy in 1918 resulted from the Spanish flu pandemic. That drop is not reflected in the child mortality data, which are available only in five-year intervals and not for 1918.

9. Jacqueline Z. M. Chan, Oona Y.-C. Lee, Ilidkó Pap, Mark Spigelman, Helen D. Donoghue, and Mark J. Pallen, "Metagenomic Analysis of Tuberculosis in a Mummy," *New England Journal of Medicine* 369 (2013): 289–290; K. I. Bos, V. J. Schuenemann, G. B. Golding, H. A. Burbano, N. Waglechner, B. K. Coombes, et al. "A Draft Genome of *Yersinia pestis* from Victims of the Black Death," *Nature* 478 (2011): 506–510; Matthias Meyer, Martin Kircher, Marie-Theres Gansauge, Heng Li, Fernando Racimo, Swapan Mallick, et al., "A High-Coverage Genome Sequence from an Archaic Denisovan Individual," *Science* 338 (2012): 222–226; Weiman Liu, Yingying Li, Gerald H. Learn, Rebecca S. Rudicell, Joel D. Robertson, Brandon F. Keele, et al., "Origin of the Human Malaria Parasite *Plasmodium falciparum* in Gorillas," *Nature* 467 (2010): 420–425.

10. For good surveys of the advances in bioarchaeology and genomics and the history of infectious diseases, see Kelly M. Harkins and Anne C. Stone, "Ancient Pathogen Genomics: Insights into Timing and Adaptation," *Journal of Human Evolution* 79 (2015): 137e149; Kristin N. Harper and George J. Armelagos, "Genomics, the Origins of Agriculture, and Our Changing Microbe-Scape: Time to Revisit Some Old Tales and Tell Some New Ones," *American Journal of Physical Anthropology* 57 (2013): 135–152.

Introduction

1. The definition of developing (or less developed) countries used in this book is taken from the UN World Population Prospects definition, which is: "all regions of Africa, Asia (except Japan), Latin America and the Caribbean plus Melanesia, Micronesia and Polynesia." UN Population Division, "Explanatory Notes," in *2015 Revision of World Population Prospects*, 2015, https://esa.un.org/poppolicy/ExplanatoryNotes.aspx.

2. Lant Pritchett, *The Rebirth of Education: Schooling Ain't Learning* (Baltimore: Brookings Institution Press, 2015), 15.

3. James C. Riley, "The Timing and Pace of Health Transitions Around the World," *Population and Development Review* 31, no. 4 (2005): 741–764; Samuel H. Preston, "Causes and Consequences of Mortality Declines in Less Developed Countries in the Twentieth Century," *Population and Economic Change in Developing Countries* (Chicago: University of Chicago Press, 1980); Rodrigo R. Soares, "On the Determinants of Mortality Reductions in the Developing World," *Population and Development Review* 33, no. 2 (2007): 247–287.

4. World Health Organization, "Global Health Observatory data," http://www.who .int/gho/hiv/en/; World Health Organization, *Global Tuberculosis Report 2017*

(Geneva: World Health Organization, 2017), 1; World Health Organization, "Global Health Estimates 2015: Estimated Deaths by Cause, 2000 and 2015," summary tables, December 2016, http://www.who.int/entity/healthinfo/global_burden_disease/GHE2015_Deaths_Global_2000_2015.xls?ua=1; World Health Organization, *Integrating Neglected Tropical Diseases into Global Health and Development* (Geneva: World Health Organization, 2017).

5. K. F. Smith, M. Goldberg, S. Rosenthal, L. Carlson, J. Chen, C. Chen, and S. Ramachandran, "2014 Global Rise in Human Infectious Disease Outbreaks," *Journal of Royal Society Interface* 11, no. 101 (2014): 20140950; K. E. Jones, N. G. Patel, M. A. Levy, A. Storeygard, D. Balk, J. L. Gitteman, and P. Daszak, "2008 Global Trends in Emerging Infectious Diseases," *Nature* 451 (2008): 990–993.

6. William H. McNeill, *Plagues and Peoples*, 3rd ed. (New York: Anchor Books and Random House, 1998), 10.

7. Douglas W. MacPherson, Brian D. Gushulak, William B. Baine, Shukal Bala, Paul O. Gubbins, Paul Holtom, and Marisel Segarra-Newnham, "Population Mobility, Globalization, and Antimicrobial Drug Resistance," *Emerging Infectious Diseases*, 15, no. 11 (2009): 1727–1732; Lance Saker et al., *Globalization and Infectious Diseases: A Review of the Linkages* (Geneva: UNICEF/UNDP/World Bank/WHO Special Program for Research and Training in Tropical Diseases, 2004).

8. Angus Deaton, "Health in an Age of Globalization" (paper presented at the Brookings Trade Forum, The Brookings Institution, Washington, DC, 2004), 3–4.

9. Ramanan Laxminarayan, Adriano Duse, Chand Wattal, Anita K. M. Zaidi, Heiman F. L. Wertheim, Nithima Sumpradit, et al., "Antibiotic Resistance—the Need for Global Solutions," *Lancet Infectious Diseases* 13, no. 12 (2013): 1057–1098.

10. Randall M. Packard, *The Making of a Tropical Disease: A Short History of Malaria* (Baltimore: Johns Hopkins University Press, 2007), 32–33, 65; Kenneth L. Gage, Thomas R. Burkot, Rebecca J. Eisen, and Edward B. Hayes, "Climate and Vectorborne Diseases," *American Journal of Preventative Medicine* 35, no. 5 (2008): 436–450; Anthony J. McMichael, "Extreme Weather Events and Infectious Disease Outbreaks," *Virulence* 6, no. 6 (2015): 543–547. The link between many infectious diseases and climate change is not linear. Research and recent modeling suggest that climate change will increase the prevalence of some pathogens in some settings but decrease them in others. Alistair Woodward, Kirk R. Smith, Diarmid Campbell-Lendrum, Dave D. Chadee, Yasushi Honda, Qiyong Liu, et al., "Climate Change and Health: On the Latest IPCC Report," *Lancet* 383, no. 9924 (2014): 1185–1189. Xiaoxu Wu, Yongmei Lu, Sen Zhou, Lifan Chen, and Bing Xu, "Impact of Climate Change on Human Infectious Diseases: Empirical Evidence and Human Adaptation," *Environment International* 86 (2016): 14–23; Anthony J. McMichael, "Globalization, Climate Change, and Human Health," *New England Journal of Medicine* 368 (2013): 1335–1343; S. Altizer, R. S. Ostfeld, P. T. Johnson, S. Kutz, and C. D. Harvell, "Climate Change and Infectious Diseases: From Evidence to a Predictive Framework," *Science* 341 (2013): 514–519.

11. A partial list of examples, arranged in alphabetical order by the author's name, follows: Ole J. Benedictow, *The Black Death, 1346–1353: The Complete History* (Woodbridge: Boydell Press, 2004); Dorothy H. Crawford, *Deadly Companions: How Microbes Shaped Our History* (Oxford: Oxford University Press, 2007); Jared Diamond, *Guns, Germs, and Steel* (New York: W. W. Norton, 1993); Kyle Harper, *The Fate of Rome: Climate, Disease, and the End of an Empire* (Princeton, NJ: Princeton University Press, 2017); Mark Harrison, *Disease and the Modern World: 1500 to the Present Day* (Cambridge: Polity Press, 2004); Donald R. Hopkins, *Princes and Peasants: Smallpox in History* (Chicago: University of Chicago Press, 1983); Steven Johnson, *The Ghost Map: The Story of London's Most Terrifying Epidemic—and How It Changed Science, Cities, and the Modern World* (New York: Riverhead Books, 2006); Arno Karlen, *Plague's Progress: A Social History of Man and Disease* (London: Phoenix Press, 2001); J. R. McNeill, *Mosquito Empires: Ecology and War in the Greater Caribbean, 1620–1914* (Cambridge: Cambridge University Press, 2010); Michael B. A. Oldstone, *Viruses, Plagues and History: Past, Present, and Future* (New York: Oxford University Press, 2010); Andrew T. Price-Smith, *Contagion and Chaos: Disease, Ecology, and National Security in the Era of Globalization* (Cambridge, MA: MIT Press, 2009); Irwin W. Sherman, *The Power of Plagues* (Washington, DC: American Society for Microbiology, 2006); Paul Slack, *The Impact of Plague in Tudor and Stuart England* (London: Routledge and Kegan Paul, 1985).

12. Zinsser, *Rats, Lice and History*, 9–10.

13. Mark Harrison, *Contagion: How Commerce Has Spread Disease* (New Haven, CT: Yale University Press, 2013).

14. Joshua Lederberg, "Medical Science, Infectious Disease, and the Unity of Humankind," *JAMA* 260, no. 5 (1988): 684–685.

15. L. S. Woolf, *International Government* (New York: Brentano's, 1916), 221.

16. David P. Fidler, *International Law and Infectious Disease* (Oxford: Clarendon Press, 1999), 6–7, 52.

17. Leviticus 13:4, 13:46, 14:8.

18. Paul Slack, "Introduction," in *Epidemics and Ideas: Essays on the Historical Perception of Pestilence*, ed. Terrence Ranger and Paul Slack (Cambridge: Cambridge University Press, 1992), 15; Dorothy Porter, "Introduction," in *The History of Public Health and the Modern State*, ed. Dorothy Porter (Amsterdam: Editions Rodopi, 1994), 2–3; Carlo M. Cipolla, *Miasmas and Disease: Public Health and the Environment in the Pre-Industrial Age* (New Haven, CT: Yale University Press, 1992).

19. Slack, *Epidemics and Ideas*, 15; John L. Brooke, *Climate Change and the Course of Global History: A Rough Journey* (Cambridge: Cambridge University Press, 2014), 424–425.

20. McNeill, *Plagues and Peoples*, 105.

21. Ron Barrett and George J. Armelagos, *An Unnatural History of Emerging Infectious Diseases* (New York: Oxford University Press, 2013), 50; Peter Baldwin, *Contagion and the State in Europe, 1830–1930* (Cambridge: Cambridge University Press, 2005), 4–6; Fidler, *International Law and Infectious Disease*, 26–28.

22. Baldwin, *Contagion and the State in Europe*, 4–6, 524–563; Porter, *History of Public Health*, 2–5, 24–25.

23. Nancy Tomes, *The Gospel of Germs: Men, Women, and the Microbe in American Life* (Cambridge, MA: Harvard University Press, 1999).

24. James C. Riley, *Rising Life Expectancy: A Global History* (New York: Cambridge University Press, 2001), 27; Stephen J. Kunitz, *The Health of Populations: General Theories and Practical Realities* (Oxford: Oxford University Press, 2007), 9–26, 45–56; Simon R. Szreter and Graham Mooney, "Urbanization, Mortality, and the New Standard of Living Debate: New Estimates of the Expectation of Life at Birth in Nineteenth-Century Cities," *Economic History Review* 51, no. 1 (1998): 84–112; Simon R. Szreter, "The Importance of Social Intervention in Britain's Mortality Decline c. 1850–1914: A Re-interpretation of the Role of Public Health," *Social History of Medicine* 1, no. 1 (1988): 1–38.

25. Thomas R. Frieden, Paula I. Fujiwara, Rita M. Washko, and Margaret A. Hamburg, "Tuberculosis in New York City—Turning the Tide," *New England Journal of Medicine* 333, no. 4 (1995): 229–233.

26. Michael Elliott, "The Age of Miracles," *Time Magazine*, Jan. 15, 2015.

27. World Bank Group, *Migration and Development: A Role for the World Bank Group* (Washington, DC: World Bank Group, 2016), 11–12.

Chapter 1: How the World Starts Getting Better

1. Given that S was a client and I have not obtained her permission to do otherwise, I use an initial instead of her name in this book.

2. UNAIDS, "AIDSinfo," http://aidsinfo.unaids.org/#data-details.

3. Peter Barron, Yogan Pillay, Tanya Doherty, Gayle Sherman, Debra Jackson, Snajana Bhardwaj, Precious Robinson, and Ameena Goga, "Eliminating Mother-to-Child HIV Transmission in South Africa," *Bulletin of the World Health Organization* 91 (2013): 70–74.

4. Patrick Martin-Tuite, "'Whose Science?' AIDS, History, and Public Knowledge in South Africa," *Intersect* 4, no. 1 (2011); Celia W. Dugger, "Study Cites Toll of AIDS Policy in South Africa," *New York Times*, Nov. 25, 2008, A1; Anthony Butler, "South Africa's HIV/AIDS, 1994–2004: How Can It Be Explained," *African Affairs* 104 (2005): 591–614.

5. Treatment Action Campaign, *Fighting for Our Lives: The History of the Treatment Action Campaign 1998–2010* (Cape Town: Treatment Action Campaign, 2010).

6. Thomas J. Bollyky, "Better, Cheaper, Faster: A More Sustainable Strategy for Treatment Access," *Stanford Journal of Law, Science and Policy* 5 (2011): 42.

7. Institute for Health Metrics and Evaluation, "Global Burden of Disease," http://www.healthdata.org/gbd.

8. George Annas, "The Right to Health and the Nevirapine Case in South Africa," *New England Journal of Medicine* 348 (2003): 750–754.

9. Dugger, "Study Cites Toll of AIDS Policy," A1.

10. Pride Chigwedere, G. R. Seage III, S. Gruskin, T. H. Lee, and M. Essex, "Estimating the Lost Benefits of Antiretroviral Drug Use in South Africa," *Journal of Acquired Immune Deficiency Syndromes* 49, no. 4 (2008): 410–415.

11. R. Burton, J. Giddy, and K. Stinson, "Prevention of Mother-to-Child Transmission in South Africa: An Ever-Changing Landscape," *Obstetric Medicine* 8, no. 1 (2015): 5–12.

12. Institute for Health Metrics and Evaluation, "Global Burden of Disease," http://www.healthdata.org/gbd.

13. Mark Nathan Cohen, *Health and the Rise of Civilization* (New Haven, CT: Yale University Press, 1989), 137.

14. Cohen, *Health and the Rise of Civilization*, 32–34, 135; Barrett and Armelagos, *Unnatural History of Emerging Infectious Diseases*, 7–8, 18–19; Mary C. Stiner, Natalie D. Munro, Todd A. Surovell, Eitan Tchernov, and Ofer Bar-Yosef, "Paleolithic Population Growth Pulses Evidenced by Small Animal Exploitation," *Science* 283 (1999): 190–194; Frank J. Fenner, "The Effects of Changing Social Organization on the Infectious Diseases of Man," in *The Impact of Civilization on the Biology of Man*, ed. Stephen Boyden (Toronto: University of Toronto Press, 1970), 48–68; Frank W. Marlowe, "Hunter-Gatherers and Human Evolution," *Evolutionary Anthropology* 14 (2005): 54–67.

15. Cohen, *Health and the Rise of Civilization*, 33–34.

16. Ian Morris, *Why the West Rules—For Now: The Patterns of History, and What They Reveal about the Future* (London: Picador Books, 2010), 346; Richard Carter and Kamini Mendis, "Evolutionary and Historical Aspects of the Burden of Malaria," *Clinical Microbiology Review* 15 (2002): 564–594; Sonia Shah, *The Fever: How Malaria Has Ruled Humankind for 500,000 Years* (London: Picador, 2010), 20–24.

17. Kristin N. Harper and George J. Armelagos, "Genomics, the Origins of Agriculture, and Our Changing Microbe-Scape: Time to Revisit Some Old Tales and Tell

Some New Ones," *American Journal of Physical Anthropology* 57 (2013): 135–152, 139; Anne C. Stone, Alicia K. Wilbur, Jane E. Buikstra, and Charlotte A. Roberts, "Tuberculosis and Leprosy in Perspective," *American Journal of Physical Anthropology* 49 (2009): 66–94; Dietmar Steverding, "The History of African Trypanosomiasis," *Parasites & Vectors* 1 (2008): 3; Ruth Hershberg, Mikhail Lipatov, Peter M Small, Hadar Sheffer, Stefan Niemann, Susanne Homolka, et al., "High Functional Diversity in Mycobacterium Tuberculosis Driven by Genetic Drift and Human Demography," *PLOS Biology* 6 (2008): e311. There is some debate as to whether the emergence of tuberculosis and leprosy may have been more recent, arising roughly four thousand years ago with the move to larger settlements. Monica H. Green, "The Globalisations of Disease," in *Human Dispersal and Species Movement: From Prehistory to the Present*, ed. Nicole Boivin, Rémy Crassard, and Michael D. Petraglia (Cambridge: Cambridge University Press, 2017), 494–520; Charlotte A. Roberts, "Old World Tuberculosis: Evidence from Human Remains with a Review of Current Research and Future Prospects," *Tuberculosis* 95, suppl. 1 (2015): S117–S121; Iñaki Comas, Mireia Coscolla, Tao Luo, Sonia Borrell, Kathryn E. Holt, Midori Kato-Maeda, et al., "Out-of-Africa Migration and Neolithic Co-expansion of Mycobacterium Tuberculosis with Modern Humans," *Nature Genetics* 45 (2013): 1176–1182; Kristen I. Bos, Kelly M. Harkins, Alexander Herbig, Mireia Coscolla, Nico Weber, Iñaki Comas, et al., "Pre-Columbian Mycobacterial Genomes Reveal Seals as a Source of New World Human Tuberculosis," *Nature* 514 (2014): 494–497; Thomas McKeown, *The Origins of Human Disease* (Cambridge, MA: Blackwell, 1988).

18. Dorian Q. Fuller, George Wilcox, and Robin G. Allaby, "Cultivation and Domestication Had Multiple Origins: Arguments against the Core Area Hypothesis for the Origins of Agriculture in the Near East," *World Archeology* 43, no. 4 (2011): 628–652; Barrett and Armelagos, *Unnatural History of Emerging Infectious Diseases*, 42.

19. James C. Scott, *Against the Grain: A Brief History of the Earliest States* (New Haven, CT: Yale University Press, 2017), 5–7; Barrett and Armelagos, *Unnatural History of Emerging Infectious Diseases*, 30; Morris, *Why the West Rules*, 107, 114–117; McKeown, *Origins of Human Disease*, 41.

20. Barrett and Armelagos, *Unnatural History of Emerging Infectious Diseases*, 31; Mark Nathan Cohen, "Introduction: Rethinking the Origins of Agriculture," *Current Anthropology* 50 (2009): 591–595. For evidence that foragers had entered into a period of extended poor health before the early transition to agriculture in the Levant, see Patricia Smith and Liora Kolska Horwitz, "Ancestors and Inheritors: Bioanthropological Perspective on the Transition to Agropastoralism in the Southern Levant," in *Ancient Health: Skeletal Indicators of Agricultural and Economic Intensification*, ed. M. N. Cohen and G. M. M. Crane-Kramer (Gainesville: University Press of Florida, 2007), 207–222.

21. Morris, *Why the West Rules*, 89, 99.

22. Cohen, *Health and the Rise of Civilization*, 39, 42, 44.

23. Vered Eshed, Avi Gopher, Ron Pinhasi, and Israel Hershkovitz, "Paleopathology and the Origin of Agriculture in the Levant," *American Journal of Physical Anthropology* 143 (2010): 121–133; Cohen, *Health and the Rise of Civilization*, 53–54, 132–137; Tim Dyson, *Population and Development: The Demographic Transition* (London: Zed Books, 2010); Barrett and Armelagos, *Unnatural History of Emerging Infectious Diseases*, 36; Angus Deaton, *The Great Escape: Health, Wealth, and the Origins of Inequality* (Princeton, NJ: Princeton University Press, 2013), 76–81; Anna Willis and Marc F. Oxenham, "The Neolithic Demographic Transition and Oral Health: The Southeast Asian Experience," *American Journal of Physical Anthropology* 152 (2013): 197–208.

24. Tania Hardy-Smith and Phillip C. Edwards, "The Garbage Crisis in Prehistory: Artifact Discard Patterns at the Early Natufian site of Wadi Hammeh 27 and the Origins of Household Refuse Disposal Strategies," *Journal of Anthropological Archaeology* 23 (2004): 253–289.

25. William L. Rathe and Cullen Murphy, *Rubbish! The Archaeology of Garbage* (Tucson: University of Arizona Press, 2001), 32; John L. Brooke, *Climate Change and the Course of Global History: A Rough Journey* (Cambridge: Cambridge University Press, 2014), 230.

26. Cohen, *Health and the Rise of Civilization*, 40; Harper and Armelagos, "Genomics, the Origins of Agriculture, and Our Changing Microbe-Scape," 139–140; Tovi Lehmann, Paula L. Marcet, Doug H. Graham, Erica R. Dahl, and J. P. Dubey, "Globalization and the Population Structure of Toxoplasma Gondii," *Proceedings of the National Academy of Sciences* 103, no. 30 (2006): 11423–11428; J. R. McNeill, *Mosquito Empires: Ecology and War in the Greater Caribbean, 1620–1914* (Cambridge: Cambridge University Press, 2010), 32.

27. Hoyt Bleakley, "Disease and Development: Evidence from Hookworm Eradication in the American South," *Quarterly Journal of Economics* 122, no. 1 (2007): 73–117.

28. Harper and Armelagos, "Genomics, the Origins of Agriculture, and Our Changing Microbe-Scape," 140; Brooke, *Climate Change and the Course of Global History*, 223; Jess A. T. Morgan, Randall J. Dejong, Grace O. Adeoye, Ebenezer D. O. Ansa, Constança S. Barbarbosa, Philippe Brémond, et al., "Origin and Diversification of the Human Parasite Schistosoma Mansoni," *Molecular Ecology* 14 (2005): 3889–3902.

29. Barrett and Armelagos, *Unnatural History of Emerging Infectious Diseases*, 40; Brooke, *Climate Change and the Course of Global History*, 221–223.

30. Harper and Armelagos, "Genomics, the Origins of Agriculture, and Our Changing Microbe-Scape," 140; Robin A. Weiss, "Animal Origins of Human Infectious Disease," *Philosophical Transactions of the Royal Society of London B: Biological Sciences* 356 (2001): 957–977, 960; Victor M. Corman, Isabella Eckerle, Ziad A. Memish, Anne M. Liljander, Ronald Dijkman, Hulda Jonsdottir, et al., "Link of a Ubiquitous Human Coronavirus to Dromedary Camels," *Proceedings of the National Academy of*

Sciences 113, no. 35 (2016): 9864–9869; Jessica M. C. Pearce-Duvet, "The Origin of Human Pathogens: Evaluating the Role of Agriculture and Domestic Animals in the Evolution of Human Disease," *Biological Reviews* 81 (2006): 369–382; Jelle Matthijnssens, "Full Genome-Based Classification of Rotaviruses Reveals a Common Origin between Human Wa-Like and Porcine Rotavirus Strains and Human DS-1-Like and Bovine Rotavirus Strains," *Journal of Virology* 82 (2008): 3204–3219.

31. Harper and Armelagos, "Genomics, the Origins of Agriculture, and Our Changing Microbe-Scape," 140; Noah Smith, R. Glyn Hewinson, Kristin Kremer, Roland Brosch, and Stephen V. Gordon, "Myths and Misconceptions: The Origin and Evolution of Mycobacterium Tuberculosis," *Nature Reviews Microbiolology* 7 (2009): 537–544; Eric P. Hoberg, Nancy L. Alkire, Alan de Queiroz, and Arlene Jones, "Out of Africa: Origins of the Taenia Tapeworms in Humans," *Proceedings of the Royal Society London B: Biological Sciences* 268 (2001): 781–787.

32. Irrigation farming also likely spread schistosomiasis, which was rampant in ancient Egypt, Japan, and China. Dorothy H. Crawford, *Deadly Companions* (Oxford: Oxford University Press, 2007), 66–73.

33. Harper and Armelagos, "Genomics, the Origins of Agriculture, and Our Changing Microbe-Scape," 138–140; Shah, *Fever*, 24–28; Kazuyuki Tanabe, Toshihiro Mita, Thibaut Jombart, Anders Eriksson, Shun Horibe, Nirianne Palacpac, et al., "*Plasmodium falciparum* Accompanied the Human Expansion Out of Africa," *Current Biology* 20 (2010): 1283–1289; Deirdre A. Joy, Xiaorong Feng, Jianbing Mu, Tetsuya Furuya, Kesinee Chotivanich, Antoniana U. Krettli, et al., "Early Origin and Recent Expansion of *Plasmodium falciparum*," *Science* 300 (2003): 318–321.

34. Pearce-Duvet, "Origin of Human Pathogens," 369–382; Igor V. Babkin and Irina N. Babkina, "A Retrospective Study of the Orthopoxvirus Molecular Evolution," *Infection, Genetics, and Evolution* 12 (2012): 1597–1604; Giovanna Morelli, Yajun Song, Camila J. Mazzoni, Mark Eppinger, Philippe Roumagnac, David M. Wagner, et al., "Phylogenetic Diversity and Historical Patterns of Pandemic Spread of *Yersinia pestis*," *Nature Genetics* 42 (2010): 1140–1143.

35. Massimo Livi-Bacci, *A Concise History of World Population*, 5th ed. (Chichester: Wiley-Blackwell, 2012), 35–41; Scott, *Against the Grain*, 6; Barrett and Armelagos, *Unnatural History of Emerging Infectious Diseases*, 36–39; Brooke, *Climate Change and the Course of Global History*, 217, 238, 270; Deaton, *Great Escape*, 80.

36. Scott, *Against the Grain*, 116–155; Seth Richardson, "Early Mesopotamia: The Presumptive State," *Past and Present* 215, no. 1 (2012): 3–49; Paul Bairoch, *Cities and Economic Development: From the Dawn of History to the Present* (Chicago: University of Chicago Press, 1988), 13, 29, 39–45.

37. William J. Bernstein, *A Splendid Exchange: How Trade Shaped the World* (New York: Grove Press, 2009), 19–28; Guillermo Algaze, *The Uruk World System: The Dynamics of*

Expansion of Early Mesopotamian Civilization, 2nd ed. (Chicago: University of Chicago Press, 2005); Scott, *Against the Grain*, 34.

38. Bernstein, *Splendid Exchange*, 19–28; Algaze, *Uruk World System*; Scott, *Against the Grain*, 34; Kyle Harper, *The Fate of Rome* (Princeton, NJ: Princeton University Press, 2017), 94–98.

39. Scott, *Against the Grain*, 100.

40. Bairoch, *Cities and Economic Development*, 26–27, 75, 223–226; Harper, *Fate of Rome*, 33–35.

41. Karen Rhea Nemet-Nejat, *Daily Life in Early Mesopotamia* (Westport, CT: Greenwood Press, 1998), 146–147.

42. Arno Karlen, *Plague's Progress: A Social History of Man and Disease* (London: Phoenix, 2001), 55.

43. Harper, *Fate of Rome*, 70–71, 82–84; Brooke, *Climate Change and the Course of Global History*, 314–316, 337; Piers D. Mitchell, "Human Parasites in the Roman World: Health Consequences of Conquering an Empire," *Parasitology* 144 (2017): 48–58; Alex Scobie, "Slums, Sanitation, and Mortality in the Roman World," *KLIO* 2 (1986): 399–433.

44. Donald R. Hopkins, *Princes and Peasants: Smallpox in History* (Chicago: University of Chicago Press, 1983), 19; Thucydides, *History of the Peloponnesian War*, trans. Rex Warner (London: Penguin, 1977), 155.

45. Most Roman historians believe the Antonine Plague was smallpox, but that conclusion has yet to be confirmed by DNA evidence. Harper, *Fate of Rome*, 102; Hopkins, *Princes and Peasants*, 21.

46. The Antonine Plague "whipsawed" around the region until at least 172 CE and reappeared in 191 CE, killing an estimated 7 or 8 million people. Another epidemic, known as the Cyprian Plague, struck in 249 CE and may have lasted fifteen years, during which time the Roman Empire effectively collapsed. Harper, *Fate of Rome*, 110–149; Brooke, *Climate Change and the Course of Global History*, 343–349.

47. David M. Wagner, Jennifer Klunk, Michaela Harbeck, Alison Devault, Nicholas Waglechner, Jason W. Sahl, et al., "*Yersinia pestis* and the Plague of Justinian 541–543 AD: A Genomic Analysis," *Lancet Infectious Diseases* 14 (2014): 319–326; Harper, *Fate of Rome*, 12, 214, 224–229.

48. Dionysios Stahakopoulos, "Population, Demography, and Disease," in *The Oxford Handbook of Byzantine Studies*, ed. Elizabeth Jeffreys, John Haldon, and Robin Cormack (New York: Oxford University Press, 2008), 310–311; Harper, *Fate of Rome*, 12, 243–245.

49. Bernstein, *Splendid Exchange*, 135–139.

50. Peter Frankopan, *The Silk Roads: A New History of the World* (New York: Vintage Books, 2017), 181; William H. McNeill, *Plagues and Peoples*, 3rd ed. (New York: Anchor Books and Random House, 1998), 176–177; Donald A. Henderson, *Smallpox: The Death of a Disease* (Amherst, NY: Prometheus Books, 2009), 39; Harrison, *Disease and Modern World*, 15–16; Karlen, *Plague's Progress*, 79–80; Bernstein, *Splendid Exchange*, 142–143; Crawford, *Deadly Companions*, 84.

51. Mark Wheelis, "Biological Warfare at the 1346 Siege of Caffa," *Emerging Infectious Diseases* 8, no. 9 (2002): 971–975.

52. There was debate over whether the Black Death was bubonic plague or another disease like anthrax, but that question now appears settled. See Lester K. Little, "Plague Historians in Lab Coats," *Past & Present* 213 (2011): 267–290; Simon Rasmissen, Morten Erik Allentoft, Kasper Nielsen, Ludovic Orlando, Martin Sikora, Karl-Göran Sjögren, et al., "Early Divergent Strains of *Yersinia pestis* in Eurasia 5,000 Years Ago," *Cell* 163 (2015): 571–582; Kristen I. Bos, Verena J. Schuenemann, G. Brian Golding, Hernán A. Burbano, Nicholas Waglechner, Brian K. Coombes, et al., "A Draft Genome of *Yersinia pestis* from Victims of the Black Death," *Nature* 478 (2011): 506–510; Yujun Cui, Chang Yub, Yanfeng Yana, Dongfang Lib, Yanjun Lia, Thibaut Jombart, et al., "Historical Variations in Mutation Rate in an Epidemic Pathogen, *Yersinia pestis*," *Proceedings of the National Academy of Science* 110 (2013): 577–582; David Herlihy, *The Black Death and the Transformation of the West* (Cambridge, MA: Harvard University Press, 1997).

53. Ole J. Benedictow, *The Black Death, 1346–1353: The Complete History* (Woodbridge: Boydell Press, 2004), 31–34. Rats also may not have been the only means by which the Black Death spread, and it remains uncertain how the disease "in an age before steam-powered (let alone jet) travel…disseminated across so much of the Eurasian and North African landscape in just a few decades." Monica H. Green, "Editor's Introduction to Pandemic Disease in the Medieval World: Rethinking the Black Death," *Medieval Globe* 1 (2014): 9–26.

54. Marchione di Coppo Stefani, *Cronaca fiorentina: Rerum Italicarum Scriptores*, vol. 30, ed. Niccolo Rodolico (Citta di Castello, 1903–1913), http://www2.iath.virginia.edu/osheim/marchione.html.

55. Agnolo di Tura del Grasso, *Cronaca Senese*, quoted in Robert S. Gottfried, *The Black Death: Natural and Human Disaster in Medieval Europe* (New York: Free Press, 1983), 45.

56. Carlo M. Cipolla, *Before the Industrial Revolution: European Society and Economy 1000–1700*, 3rd ed. (New York: W. W. Norton, 1994), 131.

57. Michael Walters Dols, *The Black Death in the Middle East* (Princeton, NJ: Princeton University Press, 1977); Bernstein, *Splendid Exchange*, 147–150.

58. Frankopan, *Silk Roads*, 184.

59. Robert Gottfried, *The Black Death: Natural and Human Disaster in Medieval Europe* (New York: Free Press, 1983), 41.

60. These advances occurred more in Northern Europe than in the then-more developed Southern parts of the continent or Egypt where the power of landlords, guilds, and other elites was more entrenched. Frankopan, *Silk Roads*, 187–188; Walter Scheidel, *The Great Leveler: Violence and the History of Inequality from the Stone Age to the Twenty-first Century* (Princeton, NJ: Princeton University Press, 2017), 300–313.

61. Ronald Findlay and Kevin O'Rourke, *Power and Plenty: Trade, War, and the World Economy in the Second Millennium* (Princeton, NJ: Princeton University Press, 2007), 111–120; Nico Voigtländer and Hans-Joachim Voth, "The Three Horsemen of Riches: Plague, War, and Urbanization in Early Modern Europe," *Review of Economic Studies* 80 (2013): 774–811.

62. Mark Harrison, *Contagion: How Commerce Has Spread Disease* (New Haven, CT: Yale University Press, 2013), 1.

63. A strain of tuberculosis existed in the pre-Columbian era in present-day Peru, probably spread there via migrating sea lions and seals. Bos et al., "Pre-Columbian Mycobacterial Genome," 494–497. Leishmaniasis, chagas, salmonella, and syphilis are believed to have existed in parts of South and Central America as well. Noble David Cook, *Born to Die: Disease and New World Conquest, 1492–1650* (Cambridge: Cambridge University Press, 1998), 17–18; David S. Jones, "Virgin Soils Revisited," *William and Mary Quarterly* 60 (2003): 703–742, 733.

64. Barrett and Armelagos, *Unnatural History of Emerging Infectious Diseases*, 42; Jared Diamond, *Guns, Germs, and Steel* (New York: W. W. Norton, 1993), 213.

65. Livi-Bacci, *Concise History of World Population*, 41–53.

66. McNeill, *Plagues and Peoples*, 210.

67. Crawford, *Deadly Companions*, 118; Åshild J. Vågene, Michael G. Campana, Nelly M. Robles García, ChristinaWarinner, Maria A. Spyrou, Aida Andrades Valtueña, et al., "*Salmonella enterica* Genomes Recovered from Victims of a Major 16th Century Epidemic in Mexico," *bioRxiv* (2017); Cook, *Born to Die*, 63–70, 86; Irwin W. Sherman, *The Power of Plagues* (Washington, DC: American Society for Microbiology Press), 193; Green, "Globalisations of Disease," 192.

68. Henderson, *Smallpox*, 41.

69. Crawford, *Deadly Companions*, 116; McNeill, *Plagues and Peoples*, 19–20; Diamond, *Guns, Germs, and Steel*, 70; Cook, *Born to Die*, 63–70.

70. Livi-Bacci, *Concise History of World Population*, 46–47; Cook, *Born to Die*, 21–59; Jones, "Virgin Soils Revisited," 720.

71. The identity of the plague(s) that struck coastal New England between 1616 and 1619 has not been fully confirmed, but many attribute it to smallpox. Henry F. Dobyns, *Their Number Became Thinned: Native American Population Dynamics in Eastern North America* (Knoxville: University of Tennessee Press, 1983); Charles C. Mann, *1491: New Revelations of the Americas before Columbus* (New York: Vintage, 2011), 106–109; Harrison, *Disease and the Modern World*, 73. But see Dean R. Snow and Kim M. Lanphear, "European Contact and Indian Depopulation in the Northeast: The Timing of the First Epidemics," *Ethnohistory* 35 (1988): 15–33.

72. Barrett and Armelagos, *Unnatural History of Emerging Infectious Diseases*, 49; Jones, "Virgin Soils Revisited," 733–742; Paul Kelton, *Epidemics and Enslavement: Biological Catastrophe in the Native Southeast, 1492–1715* (Lincoln: University of Nebraska Press, 2007).

73. Henderson, *Smallpox*, 42.

74. Elizabeth A. Fenn, "Biological Warfare in Eighteenth-Century North America: Beyond Jeffery Amherst," *Journal of American History* 86, no. 4 (2000): 1552–1580.

75. Quoted in Margaret Humphreys, *Malaria: Poverty, Race, and Public Health in the United States* (Baltimore: Johns Hopkins University Press, 2001), 68.

76. Harrison, *Disease and the Modern World*, 79; Crawford, *Deadly Companions*, 118–121.

77. McNeill, *Mosquito Empires*, 4, 33, 40–41, 51.

78. See Claude Quetel, *History of Syphilis* (Baltimore: Johns Hopkins University Press, 1992); Barrett and Armelagos, *Unnatural History of Emerging Infectious Diseases*, 46; Crawford, *Deadly Companions*, 123–130.

79. Giovanni Berlinguer, "Globalization and Global Health," *International Journal of Health Services* 29, no. 3 (1999): 579–595; Giovanni Berlinguer, "The Interchange of Disease and Health between the Old and New Worlds," *American Journal of Public Health* 82, no. 10 (1992): 1407–1413; Stephen Morse, "Global Microbial Traffic and the Interchange of Disease," *American Journal of Public Health* 82, no. 10 (1992): 1326–1327; Riley, *Rising Life Expectancy*, 82–83; Emmanuel Le Roy Ladurie, *Un Concept: L'Unification Microbienne due Monde* (Geneva: Société Suisse d'Histoire, 1973), 4.

80. Bairoch, *Cities and Economic Development*, 130–132; Robert H. Bates, *Prosperity and Violence: The Political Economy of Development* (New York: W. W. Norton, 2001), 51–53.

81. Robert Woods, "Urbanization in Europe and China during the Second Millennium: A Review of Urbanism and Demography," *International Journal of Population Geography* 9, no. 3 (2003): 215–227.

82. Cohen, *Health and the Rise of Civilization*, 140.

83. Genesis 3: 17–19. George Armelagos and Kristin Harper also point out that the Ramayana, one of India's great epics, takes a similarly dim view of agriculture. Harper and Armelagos, "Genomics, the Origins of Agriculture, and Our Changing Microbe-Scape," 135.

84. Jared Diamond, "The Worst Mistake in the History of the Human Race," *Discover*, May 1987, 86.

85. Steven Pinker, *The Better Angels of Our Nature: Why Violence Has Declined* (London: Penguin, 2011), 43–56. Recent paleoanthropological studies found evidence of decreased skull trauma with the transition to agriculture in the Levant region. Eshed et al., "Paleopathology and the Origin of Agriculture," 121–133.

86. Abdel R. Omran, "The Epidemiologic Transition: A Theory of Epidemiology of Population Change," *Milbank Quarterly* 49, no. 4 (Oct. 1971): 509–538. Some more recent estimates suggest Roman life expectancy might have been a bit higher, roughly 27 years. Harper, *Fate of Rome*, 73; Clio Infra, "Life Expectancy at Birth (Total)—UK," 2014, https://www.clio-infra.eu/datasets/Indicators/LifeExpectancyat BirthTotal.html.

87. Javier Birchenall, "Economic Development and the Escape from High Mortality," *World Development* 35, no. 4 (April 2007): 543–568.

88. Thomas McKeown, *The Origins of Human Disease* (Cambridge, MA: Blackwell, 1988); Robert William Fogel, *The Escape from Hunger and Premature Death, 1700–2100: Europe, America, and the Third World* (Cambridge: Cambridge University Press, 2004).

89. Deaton, *Great Escape*, 82.

90. Simon Szreter, *Health and Wealth: Studies in History and Policy* (Rochester: University of Rochester Press, 2007), 210–212.

91. Livi-Bacci, *Concise History of World Population*, 72; Deaton, *Great Escape*, 92–93.

92. Thomas Malthus, "Population," in *Supplement to the Fourth, Fifth, and Sixth Editions of the Encylopaedia Britannica* (Edinburgh: Arichbald Constable, 1824), 322.

93. Charles Dickens, *A Christmas Carol* (London: William Heinemann, 1906), 8–9.

94. Harrison, *Disease and the Modern World*, 111.

95. J. N. Hays, *The Burdens of Disease: Epidemics and Human Response in Western History* (New Brunswick, NJ: Rutgers University Press, 1998), 245; Marie-France Morel, "The Care of Children: The Influence of Medical Innovation and Medical Institutions on Infant Mortality, 1750–1914," in *The Decline of Mortality*, ed. Roger Schofield, David Reher, and Alain Bideau (Oxford: Oxford University Press, 1991), 196–219.

96. Joel Mokyr, "Technological Progress and the Decline of European Mortality," *American Economic Review* 83, no. 2 (May 1993): 324–330.

97. Harrison, *Disease and the Modern World*, 111–112; Dorothy Porter, *Health, Civilization, and the State: A History of Public Health from Ancient to Modern Times* (New York: Routledge Books, 1999), 115–116.

98. Harrison, *Disease and the Modern World*, 61.

99. Anna Davin, "Imperialism and Motherhood," *History Workshop*, no. 5 (Oxford: Oxford University Press, 1978), 9–58. See also George Rosen, *A History of Public Health* (Baltimore: Johns Hopkins University Press, 1991), 54–55.

100. Harrison, *Disease and the Modern World*, 111.

101. Samuel Cohn and Ruth Kutalek, "Historical Parallels, Ebola Virus Disease and Cholera: Understanding Community Distrust and Social Violence with Epidemics," *PLOS Currents Outbreaks* (Jan. 26, 2016): 1; Geoffrey Gill, Sean Burrell, and Jody Brown, "Fear and Frustration—the Liverpool Cholera Riots of 1832," *Lancet* 358 (2001): 233–237; Sean Burrell and Geoffrey Gill, "The Liverpool Cholera Epidemic of 1832 and Anatomical Dissection—Medical Mistrust and Civil Unrest," *Journal of the History of Medicine and Allied Sciences* 60, no. 4 (2005): 478–498; Peter Baldwin, *Contagion and the State in Europe, 1830–1930* (Cambridge: Cambridge University Press, 1999), 47, 62, 115–116; Charles E. Rosenberg, *The Cholera Years: The United States in 1832, 1849, and 1866* (Chicago: University of Chicago Press, 1962), 119; Frank M. Snowden, *Naples in the Time of Cholera, 1884–1911* (Cambridge: Cambridge University Press, 1995), 146–154.

102. Christopher Hamlin, *Cholera: The Biography* (Oxford: Oxford University Press, 2009), 105–120; Richard J. Evans, "Epidemics and Revolutions: Cholera in Nineteenth-Century Europe," in *Epidemics and Ideas: Essays on the Historical Perception of Pestilence*, ed. T. Ranger and P. Slack (Cambridge: Cambridge University Press, 1992), 149–173.

103. Deaton, *Great Escape*, 96; James C. Riley, "The Timing and Pace of Health Transitions around the World," *Population and Development Review* 31 (2005): 741–764.

104. Harrison, *Disease and the Modern World*, 109–117; Porter, *Health, Civilization, and the State*, 98–99, 102, 108–109, 119; John Duffy, *The Sanitarians: A History of American Public Health* (Urbana: University of Illinois Press), 44, 62, 71, 84; Gill, Burrell, and Brown, "Fear and Frustration"; Geoffrey Gill, "Cholera and Public Health Reform in Nineteenth-Century Wallasey," *Transactions of the Historic Society of Lancashire and Cheshire* 150 (2001): 57–95; William Easterly, *The Tyranny of Experts: Economists, Dictators, and the Forgotten Rights of the Poor* (New York: Basic Books, 2014).

105. Harrison, *Disease and the Modern World*, 114.

106. Edward Glaeser, *Triumph of the City: How Our Greatest Invention Makes Us Richer, Smarter, Greener, Healthier, and Happier* (London: Pan Books, 2012), 99–104; Porter, *Health, Civilization, and the State*, 147–155; Rosenberg, *Cholera Years*, 17–19, 82–98; Duffy, *The Sanitarians*, 89–91.

107. David Cutler and Grant Miller, "The Role of Public Health Improvements in Health Advances: The Twentieth-Century United States," *Demography* 42, no. 1 (Feb. 2005): 1–22.

108. Riley, "Timing and Pace of Health Transitions," 741–764; Soares, "On the Determinants of Mortality Reductions," 247–287.

109. Richard A. Easterlin, "How Beneficent Is the Market? A Look at the Modern History of Mortality," *European Review of Economic History* 3, no. 3 (1999): 257–294; Simon Szreter, "Economic Growth, Disruption, Deprivation, Disease and Death: On the Importance of the Politics of Public Health for Development," *Population and Development Review* 23, no. 4 (1997): 693–728; Stephen J. Kunitz and Stanley L. Engerman, "The Ranks of Death: Secular Trends in Income and Mortality," *Health Transition Review* 2, supplement, *Historical Epidemiology and the Health Transition* (1992): 26–46.

110. Harrison, *Disease and the Modern World*, 2, 6.

111. Baldwin, *Contagion and the State in Europe*, 524–563.

112. Baldwin, *Contagion and the State in Europe*, 345.

113. Ambe J. Njoh, "Colonization and Sanitation in Urban Africa: A Logistics Analysis of the Availability of Central Sewerage Systems as a Function of Colonialism," *Habitat International* 38 (2013): 207–213; Ambe J. Njoh and Fenda Akiwumi, "The Impact of Colonization on Access to Improved Water and Sanitation Facilities in African Cities," *Cities* 28 (2011): 452–460; Sheldon Watts, *Epidemics and History: Disease, Power, and Imperialism* (New Haven, CT: Yale University Press, 1997), xv–xvi.

114. John Sender, "Africa's Economic Performance: Limitations of the Current Consensus," *Journal of Economic Perspectives* 13 (1999): 89–114; Alexander E. Kentikelenis, Thomas H. Stubbs, and Lawrence P. King, "Structural Adjustment and Public Spending on Health: Evidence from IMF Programs in Low-Income Countries," *Social Science and Medicine* 126 (2015): 169–176.

115. David N. Weil, "A Review of Angus Deaton's *The Great Escape: Health, Wealth, and the Origins of Inequality*," *Journal of Economic Literature* 53, no. 1 (March 2015): 102–114.

116. Seema Jayachandran, Adriana Lleras-Muney, and Kimberly V. Smith, "Modern Medicine and the 20th Century Decline in Mortality: Evidence on the Impact of Sulfa Drugs" (working paper, The National Bureau of Economic Research, no. 15089, June 2009), 5.

117. "Vital Statistics," Editorial, *Nature* 494 (Feb. 19, 2013): 281.

118. Max Roser, "Life Expectancy," *Our World in Data*, 2006, https://ourworldindata.org/life-expectancy; Mattias Lindgren, Klara Johansson, and Ola Rosling, "Life Expectancy (Years)," Gapminder, 2016, https://www.gapminder.org/data/.

119. Deaton, *Great Escape*, 114–119.

Chapter 2: Diseases of Conquest and Colony

1. William H. Foege, *House on Fire: The Fight to Eradicate Smallpox* (Berkeley: University of California Press, 2011), 188.

2. Peter Gill, *Famine and Foreigners: Ethiopia since Live Aid* (Oxford: Oxford University Press, 2010), 12.

3. Abhijit Banerjee and Ester Duflo, *Poor Economics: A Radical Rethinking of the Way to Fight Global Poverty* (New York: PublicAffairs, 2011), 19.

4. Institute for Health Metrics and Evaluation, "Ethiopia Country Profile," http://www.healthdata.org/ethiopia.

5. Richard Downie, "Sustaining Improvements to Public Health in Ethiopia" (Washington, DC: Center for Strategic and International Studies, March 2016), 3.

6. Institute for Health Metrics and Evaluation, "Global Burden of Disease," http://www.healthdata.org/gbd.

7. UN Population Division, *2017 Revision of World Population Prospects*, 2017, https://esa.un.org/unpd/wpp/.

8. Institute for Health Metrics and Evaluation, "Global Burden of Disease," http://www.healthdata.org/gbd.

9. Dengue fever is the most significant exception, with deaths from this disease increasing from 19, 547 in 2005 to 37,780 in 2016. Ebola caused 11,308 deaths between December 2013 and March 2016. Zika causes few deaths, but disability associated with infection from the virus increased since 2014. Death and disability from chagas, leprosy, and trachoma globally have stayed essentially flat since 2005, but the rate of fatalities from those diseases has declined since the population increased over that time. See Institute for Health Metrics and Evaluation, "Global Burden of Disease," http://www.healthdata.org/gbd.

10. UN Population Division, "2017 Revision of World Population Prospects."

11. World Bank Group, "World Bank Forecasts Global Poverty to Fall Below 10% for First Time; Major Hurdles Remain in Goal to End Poverty by 2030," Oct. 4, 2015, http://www.worldbank.org/en/news/press-release/2015/10/04/world-bank-forecasts-global-poverty-to-fall-below-10-for-first-time-major-hurdles-remain-in-goal-to-end-poverty-by-2030.

12. Mark Harrison, *Contagion: How Commerce Has Spread Disease* (New Haven, CT: Yale University Press, 2013), 73–79.

13. David P. Fidler, "The Globalization of Public Health: The First 100 Years of International Health Diplomacy," *Bulletin of the World Health Organization* 79, no. 9 (2001): 842–849.

14. Elizabeth Fee and Theodore M. Brown, "100 Years of the Pan American Health Organization," *American Journal of Public Health* 92 (2002): 1888–1889.

15. Anne-Emmanuelle Birn, Yogan Pillay, and Tim H. Holtz, *Textbook of Global Health* (New York: Oxford University Press, 2016), 26.

16. David P. Fidler, *International Law and Infectious Disease* (Oxford: Clarendon Press, 1999), 26–57.

17. Igor V. Babkin and Irina V. Babkina, "The Origin of the Variola Virus," *Viruses* 7 (2015): 1100–1112; Igor V. Babkin and Irina N. Babkina, "A Retrospective Study of the Orthopoxvirus Molecular Evolution," *Infection, Genetics, and Evolution* 12 (2012): 1597–1604; Kristin N. Harper and George J. Armelagos, "Genomics, the Origins of Agriculture, and Our Changing Microbe-Scape: Time to Revisit Some Old Tales and Tell Some New Ones," *American Journal of Physical Anthropology* 57 (2013): 135–152, 139; Yu Li, Darin S. Carroll, Shea N. Gardner, Matthew C. Walsh, Elizabeth A. Vitalis, and Inger K. Damon, "On the Origin of Smallpox: Correlating Variola Phylogenics with Historical Smallpox Records," *Proceedings of the National Academy of Science* 104 (2007): 15787–15792; Kyle Harper, *The Fate of Rome* (Princeton, NJ: Princeton University Press, 2017), 91–92; Donald A. Henderson, *Smallpox: The Death of a Disease* (Amherst, NY: Prometheus Books, 2009), 37.

18. Sherman, *Power of Plagues*, 193; Monica H. Green, "The Globalisations of Disease," in *Human Dispersal and Species Movement: From Prehistory to the Present*, ed. Nicole Boivin, Rémy Crassard, and Michael D. Petraglia (Cambridge: Cambridge University Press, 2017), 506–510.

19. Crawford, *Deadly Companions*, 109; Sherman, *Power of Plagues*, 206.

20. Richard Preston, *The Demon in the Freezer: A True Story* (New York: Ballantine Books, 2003), 35.

21. American Public Health Association, *Control of Communicable Diseases Manual*, 20th ed., ed. David L. Heymann (Washington, DC: APHA Press, 2015), 562.

22. Henderson, *Smallpox*, 39.

23. Oscar Reiss, *Medicine and the American Revolution: How Diseases and Their Treatments Affected the Continental Army* (Jefferson, NC: MacFarland, 1998), 95–98.

24. John Rhodes, *The End of Plagues: The Global Battle against Infectious Disease* (New York: Palgrave Macmillan, 2013), 28.

25. Michael B. A. Oldstone, *Viruses, Plagues and History: Past, Present, and Future* (Oxford: Oxford University Press: 2010), 67–68.

26. Henderson, *Smallpox*, 39; Dorothy H. Crawford, *Deadly Companions* (Oxford: Oxford University Press, 2007), 110–111.

27. Livia Schrick, Simon H. Tausch, P. Wojciech Dabrowski, Clarissa R. Damaso, José Esparza, Andreas Nitsche, et al., "An Early American Smallpox Vaccine Based on Horsepox," *New England Journal of Medicine* 377 (2017): 1491–1492.

28. Rhodes, *End of Plagues*, 56–63.

29. Henderson, *Smallpox*, 47–48.

30. Rhodes, *End of Plagues*, 53; Stephen Coss, *The Fever of 1721: The Epidemic That Revolutionized Medicine and American Politics* (New York: Simon and Schuster, 2016), 276; John Duffy, *The Sanitarians: A History of American Public Health* (Champaign: University of Illinois Press, 1992), 56.

31. Harrison, *Disease and the Modern World*; Angus Deaton, *The Great Escape: Health, Wealth, and the Origins of Inequality* (Princeton, NJ: Princeton University Press, 2013).

32. P. Baldwin, *Contagion and the State in Europe, 1830–1930* (Cambridge: Cambridge University Press, 1999), 293.

33. Erwin Chemerinsky and Michele Goodwin, "Compulsory Vaccination Laws are Constitutional," *Northwestern University Law Review* 110, no. 3 (2016): 596. In *Jacobson v. Massachusetts*, 197 U.S. 11, 27 (1905), the US Supreme Court held that state compulsory vaccination laws are constitutional when they are "necessary for the public health or the public safety." The Supreme Court has affirmed the constitutionality of state compulsory vaccination laws in subsequent cases such as *Zucht v. King*, 260 U.S. 174, 177 (1922), which also upheld childhood vaccination requirements for entrance to public schools.

34. Oldstone, *Viruses, Plagues and History*, 17; Stanford T. Shulman, "The History of Pediatric Infectious Disease," *Pediatric Research* 55 (2004): 163–176.

35. Rhodes, *End of Plagues*, 62–63.

36. Sarah A. Tishkoff, Robert Varkonyi, Nelie Cahinhinan, Salem Abbes, George Argyropoulos, Giovanni Destro-Bisol, et al., "Haplotype Diversity and Linkage Disequilibrium at Human G6PD: Recent Origin of Alleles That Confer Malarial Resistance," *Science* 293 (2001): 455–462; Harper and Armelagos, "Genomics, the Origins of Agriculture, and Our Changing Microbe-Scape," 139.

37. Quoted in epigraph of Sonia Shah, *The Fever: How Malaria Has Ruled Humankind for 500,000 Years* (London: Picador, 2010).

38. Herbert S. Klein, *The Atlantic Slave Trade* (Cambridge: Cambridge University Press, 1999), 68.

39. Richard Holmes, *The Age of Wonder* (New York: Pantheon Books, 2008), 220–234.

40. McNeill, *Plagues and Peoples*, 105.

41. Andrew McIlwaine Bell, *Mosquito Soldiers: Malaria, Yellow Fever, and the Course of the American Civil War* (Baton Rouge: Louisiana State University Press, 2010), 2; Robert F. Reilly, "Medical and Surgical Care during the American Civil War, 1861–1865," *Baylor University Medical Center Proceedings* 29, no. 2 (April 2016): 138–142.

42. Bernard J. Brabin, "Malaria's Contribution to World War One—The Unexpected Adversary," *Malaria Journal* 13 (2014): 497.

43. Paul Reiter, "From Shakespeare to Defoe: Malaria in England in the Little Ice Age," *Emerging Infectious Diseases* 6, no. 1 (2000): 1–11.

44. Margaret Humphreys, *Malaria: Poverty, Race, and Public Health in the United States* (Baltimore: Johns Hopkins University Press, 2001), 74.

45. Humphreys, *Malaria*, 89–90.

46. Humphreys, *Malaria*, 140.

47. World Health Organization, "Malaria Fact Sheet," updated Nov. 2017, http://www.who.int/mediacentre/factsheets/fs094/en/.

48. Charles Kenny, *Getting Better: Why Global Development Is Succeeding—and How We Can Improve the World Even More* (New York: Basic Books, 2012), 123.

49. Catherine Mark and José G. Rigau-Pérez, "The World's First Immunization Campaign: The Spanish Smallpox Vaccine Expedition, 1803–1813," *Bulletin of the History of Medicine* 83, no. 1 (2009): 63–94.

50. Carlos Franco-Paredes, Lorena Lammoglia, and José Ignacio Santos-Preciado, "The Spanish Royal Philanthropic Expedition to Bring Smallpox Vaccination to the New World and Asia in the 19th Century," *Clinical Infectious Diseases* 41 (2005): 1285–1289; Xavier Bosch, "Review: The Spanish Royal Philanthropic Expedition: The Round-the-World Voyage of the Smallpox Vaccine 1803–1810," *Lancet Infectious Diseases* 4 (2004): 59.

51. David Arnold, "Smallpox and Colonial Medicine in Nineteenth-Century India," in *Imperial Medicine and Indigenous Societies*, ed. David Arnold (Manchester: Manchester University Press, 1988), 45–65.

52. Mark and Rigau-Pérez, "World's First Immunization Campaign," 63–94.

53. Henderson, *Smallpox*, 51–53.

54. Arnold, "Smallpox and Colonial Medicine," 45–65.

55. Sanjoy Bhattacharya, Mark Harrison, and Michael Worboys, *Fractured States: Smallpox, Public Health and Vaccination Policy in British India 1800–1947* (Himayat-nagar: Orient Blackswan, 2005), 3; Arnold, "Smallpox and Colonial Medicine," 48.

56. Enrique Soto-Pérez-de-Celis, "The Royal Philanthropic Expedition of the Vaccine: A Landmark in the History of Public Health," *Postgraduate Medical Journal* 84 (2008): 509–602.

57. Franco-Parades et al., "Spanish Royal Philanthropic Expedition," 1285–1286.

58. Birn, Pillay, and Holtz, *Textbook of Global Health*, 26; Bhattacharya, Harrison, and Worboys, *Fractured States*.

59. Packard, *Making of a Tropical Disease*, 3–4, 84–100.

60. Milton I. Roemer, "Internationalism in Medicine and Public Health," in *The History of Public Health and the Modern State*, ed. Dorothy Porter (Amsterdam: Editions Rodopi, 1994), 403–406.

61. Harrison, *Disease and the Modern World*, 134.

62. L. J. Bruce-Chwatt, "Alphonse Laveran's Discovery 100 Years Ago and Today's Global Fight against Malaria," *Journal of the Royal Society of Medicine* 74 (1981): 531–536; Harrison, *Disease and the Modern World*, 133–136.

63. Randall M. Packard, *A History of Global Health: Interventions into the Lives of Other Peoples* (Baltimore: Johns Hopkins University Press, 2016), 21; Humphreys, *Malaria*, 69.

64. McNeill, *Mosquito Empires*, 312.

65. John Farley, *To Cast Out Disease: A History of the International Health Division of the Rockefeller Foundation (1913–1951)* (Oxford: Oxford University Press, 2004), 8–17; Crawford, *Deadly Companions*, 122–123.

66. Packard, *History of Global Health*, 57–59.

67. Shah, *Fever*, 98–99.

68. Malcolm Gladwell, "The Mosquito Killer," *New Yorker*, July 2, 2001, http://www .newyorker.com/magazine/2001/07/02/the-mosquito-killer.

69. Martin Hadlow, "The Mosquito Network: American Military Broadcasting in the South-West Pacific, 1944–1946," in *The Military and the Media: The 2008 Chief of Army Military History Conference*, ed. Peter Dennis and Jeffrey Grey (Canberra: Australian Military History Publications, 2009), 74–95.

70. US Army Medical Department, *United States Army Preventive Medicine in World War II*, vol. 6, *Malaria*, ed. John Boyd Coates Jr., Ebbe Curtis Hoff, and Phebe M. Hoff (Washington, DC: US Army, 1963), table 12.

71. Packard, *History of Global Health*, 108; Fiammetta Rocco, *The Miraculous Fever-Tree: Malaria and the Quest for a Cure That Changed the World* (New York: Harper-Collins, 2003), 77.

72. Charles M. Wheeler, "Control of Typhus in Italy 1943–44 by Use of DDT," *American Journal of Public Health* 46 (1946): 119–129; Frank Snowden, *The Conquest of Italy: 1900–1962* (New Haven, CT: Yale University Press, 2006); 199; John M. Hutzel, "Insect Control for the Marines," *Scientific Monthly* 62 (1946): 417–420.

73. "Public to Receive DDT Insecticide," *New York Times*, July 27, 1945, 17.

74. Europe was not declared entirely free of malaria cases until 1975. World Health Organization, "History of Malaria Elimination in Europe," April 20, 2016, http://www.euro.who.int/__data/assets/pdf_file/0003/307272/Facsheet-malaria-elimination.pdf.

75. New vaccines and drugs for influenza, plague, tuberculosis, and pneumococcal pneumonia were discovered during the war and production of prewar drugs such as penicillin was dramatically increased. Packard, *History of Global Health*, 108.

76. Packard, *History of Global Health*, 113.

77. Packard, *History of Global Health*, 152.

78. Cost of the program in 1967 is calculated in 2016 dollars, using an average annual inflation rate of 4.11 percent from the US Bureau of Labor Statistics. Randall Packard, *The Making of a Tropical Disease: A Short History of Malaria* (Baltimore: Johns Hopkins University Press, 2007), 147; Shah, *Fever*, 216; Harrison, *Disease and the Modern World*, 181–182; Packard, *History of Global Health*, 156–158.

79. Henderson, *Smallpox: The Death of a Disease*, 87–88; Packard, *History of Global Health*, 154.

80. The White House, "Statements by the President on Announcing U.S. Support for an International Program to Eradication Smallpox," May 18, 1965, http://www.presidency.ucsb.edu/ws/?pid=26977; Nancy Stepan, *Eradication: Ridding the World of Diseases Forever?* (Ithaca, NY: Cornell University Press, 2011), 208–213.

81. Laurie Garrett, *The Coming Plague: Newly Emerging Diseases in a World Out of Balance* (New York: Penguin, 1995), 46.

82. World Health Organization, *The Global Eradication of Smallpox: Final Report of the Global Commission for the Certification of Smallpox Eradication* (Geneva, 1980), annexes 16–17.

83. World Health Organization, A33/VR/8, *Declaration of Global Eradication of Smallpox*, Thirty-third World Health Assembly, May 8, 1980, http://apps.who.int/iris/bitstream/10665/155528/1/WHA33_R3_eng.pdf.

84. World Health Organization Maximizing Positive Synergies Collaborative Group, "An Assessment of Interactions between Global Health Initiatives and Country Health Systems," *Lancet*, 373, no. 9681 (June 20, 2009): 2137–2169.

85. Farley, *To Cast Out Disease*, 4–7.

86. Farley, *To Cast Out Disease*, 31.

87. Sanjoy Battacharya, *Expunging Variola: The Control and Eradication of Smallpox in India, 1947–1977* (New Delhi: New Orient Longman Printing, 2006), 163–252; Stepan, *Eradication*, 212–215.

88. Henderson, *Smallpox*, 89-90.

89. James C. Riley, *Low Income, Social Growth, and Good Health: A History of Twelve Countries* (Berkeley: University of California Press, 2008), 111–112.

90. John C. Caldwell, "Routes to Low Mortality in Poor Countries," *Population and Development Review* 12, no. 2 (June 1986): 171–220.

91. These average annual gains in life expectancy occurred over 1947 to 1958. Mattias Lindgren, Klara Johansson, and Ola Rosling, "Life Expectancy (Years)," Gapminder, 2016, https://www.gapminder.org/data/; Davidson R. Gwatkin, "Indications of Change in Developing Country Mortality Trends: The End of an Era?" *Population and Development Review* 6, no. 4 (1980): 615–644.

92. Riley, *Low Income, Social Growth, and Good Health*, 109–114; David Cutler, Angus Deaton, and Adriana Lleras-Muney, "The Determinants of Mortality," *Journal of Economic Perspectives* 20, no. 3 (2006): 97–120.

93. James C. Riley, "The Timing and Pace of Health Transitions around the World," *Population and Development Review* 31 (2005): 741–764.

94. Samuel H. Preston, "Causes and Consequences of Mortality Declines in Less Developed Countries in the Twentieth Century," in *Population and Economic Change in Developing Countries*, ed. Richard A. Easterlin (Chicago: University of Chicago Press, 1980), 300.

95. Rodrigo R. Soares, "On the Determinants of Mortality Reductions in the Developing World," *Population and Development Review* 33, no. 2 (2007): 247–287; David M. Bishai, Robert Cohen, Y. Natalia Alfonso, Taghreed Adam, Shyama Kuruvilla, and Julian Schweitzer, "Factors Contributing to Maternal and Child Mortality Reductions in 146 Low- and Middle-Income Countries between 1990 and 2010," *PLOS ONE* 11, no. 1 (2016): e0144908.

96. Packard, *History of Global Health*, 216.

97. UNAIDS, "Fact Sheet—Latest Statistics on the Status of the AIDS Epidemic," modified Nov. 2016, http://www.unaids.org/sites/default/files/media_asset/UNAIDS _FactSheet_en.pdf.

98. UNAIDS, "Fact Sheet"; AIDSinfo, "Indicators," http://aidsinfo.unaids.org.

99. Carsten Fink and Keith E. Maskus, *Intellectual Property and Development: Lessons from Recent Economic Research* (Washington, DC, and New York: The World Bank and Oxford University Press, 2005).

100. Ellen 't Hoen, Jonathan Berger, Alexandra Calmy, and Suerie Moon, "Driving a Decade of Change: HIV/AIDS, Patents and Access to Medicines for All," *Journal of the International AIDS Society* 14, no. 15 (March 27, 2011): 3.

101. Institute for Health Metrics and Evaluation, *Financing Global Health 2015: Development Assistance Steady on the Path to New Global Goals* (Seattle: Institute for Health Metrics and Evaluation, 2016).

102. Policy Cures, "G-Finder 2015," http://policycures.org/g-finder2015.html.

103. Felicia M. Knaul, Julie R. Gralow, Rifat Atun, and Afsan Bhadelia, eds., *Closing the Cancer Divide: An Equity Imperative* (Boston: Harvard Global Equity Initiative, 2011), 221.

104. World Health Organization, "Antiretroviral Therapy (ART) Coverage among All Age Groups," http://www.who.int/gho/hiv/epidemic_response/ART_text/en/.

105. John Donnelly, "The President's Emergency Plan for AIDS Relief: How George W. Bush and Aides Came to 'Think Big' on Battling HIV," *Health Affairs* 31 (2012): 1389–1396.

106. Harley Feldbaum, Kelley Lee, and Joshua Michaud, "Global Health and Foreign Policy," *Epidemiologic Reviews* 32, no. 1 (2010): 82–92.

107. Thomas J. Bollyky, "Access for Drugs for Treatment of Noncommunicable Diseases," *PLOS Medicine* 10, no. 7 (July 23, 2013).

108. Institute for Health Metrics and Evaluation, *Financing Global Health 2015*; Institute for Health Metrics and Evaluation, "Global Burden of Disease," http://www.healthdata.org/gbd.

109. Chelsea Clinton and Devi Sridhar, *Governing Global Health: Who Runs the World and Why?* (New York: Oxford University Press, 2017), 11, 210.

110. Institute for Health Metrics and Evaluation, *Financing Global Health 2013*, 61–66.

111. Data use the World Bank definition of sub-Saharan Africa, which includes forty-eight countries. Data are from Institute for Health Metrics and Evaluation, *Financing Global Health 2016*.

112. Institute for Health Metrics and Evaluation, *Financing Global Health 2016*; World Bank DataBank, "Population (Total)," http://data.worldbank.org/indicator/SP.POP.TOTL.

113. Joseph Dieleman and Michael Hanlon, "Measuring the Displacement and Replacement of Government Heath Expenditure," *Health Economics* 23, no. 2 (Feb. 2014): 129–140.

114. Packard, *History of Global Health,* 5.

115. PriceWaterhouseCoopers, "From Vision to Decision: Pharma 2020," Nov. 2012, http://download.pwc.com/ie/pubs/2012_pharma_2020.pdf.

116. R. Laxminarayan, A. Duse, C. Wattal, A. K. Zaidi, H. F. Wertheim, N. Sumpradit, et al., "Antibiotic Resistance—The Need for Global Solutions," *Lancet Infectious Diseases* 13, no. 12 (Dec. 2013): 1057–1098; Gardiner Harris, "Superbugs' Kill India's Babies and Pose an Overseas Threat," *New York Times,* Dec. 4, 2014, https://www.nytimes.com/2014/12/04/world/asia/superbugs-kill-indias-babies-and-pose-an-overseas-threat.html?_r=0.

117. Landon Thomas Jr., "An Investor's Plan to Transplant Private Health Care in Africa," *New York Times,* Oct. 9, 2016, https://www.nytimes.com/2016/10/09/business/dealbook/an-investors-plan-to-transplant-private-health-care-in-africa.html.

118. Hubert Trowell and Denis Burkitt, eds., *Western Diseases: Their Emergence and Prevention* (Cambridge, MA: Harvard University Press, 1981), 4–8, 14.

119. Mitchell E. Daniels Jr., Thomas E. Donilon, Thomas J. Bollyky, and Christopher M. Tuttle, *The Emerging Global Health Crisis: Noncommunicable Diseases in Low- and Middle-Income Countries,* Independent Task Force Report no. 72 (New York: Council on Foreign Relations Press, 2014).

120. Thomas J. Bollyky, Tara Templin, Matthew Cohen, and Joseph L. Dieleman, "Lower-Income Countries That Face the Most Rapid Shift in Noncommunicable Disease Burden Are Also the Least Prepared," *Health Affairs* 36 (2017): 1866–1875.

121. Marie Ng, Tom Fleming, Margaret Robinson, Blake Thomson, Nicholas Graetz, Christopher Margono, et al., "Global, Regional, and National Prevalence of Overweight and Obesity in Children and Adults during 1980–2013: A Systematic Analysis for the Global Burden of Disease Study 2013," *Lancet* 384, no. 9945 (2014): 766–781.

122. Council on Foreign Relations, "The Emerging Crisis: Noncommunicable Diseases," 2014, http://www.cfr.org/diseases-noncommunicable/ncds-interactive/p33802.

123. David S. Reher, "Economic and Social Implications of the Demographic Transition," *Population and Development Review* 37 (2011): 11–33.

124. Institute for Health Metrics and Evaluation, "Global Burden of Disease," 2015, http://www.healthdata.org/gbd.

125. Thomas J. Bollyky, Tara Templin, Caroline Andridge, and Joseph L. Dieleman, "Understanding the Relationships between Non-Communicable Diseases, Unhealthy Lifestyles, and Country Wealth," *Health Affairs* 34, no. 9 (2015): 1464–1471.

126. Reher, "Economic and Social Implications."

127. Institute for Health Metrics and Evaluation, "Global Burden of Disease," 2015, http://www.healthdata.org/gbd.

128. UN Population Division, "2017 Revision of World Population Prospects."

129. Bollyky et al., "Lower-Income Countries That Face the Most Rapid Shift," 1866–1875.

130. Toulant Muka, David Imo, Veronica Colpani, Layal Chaker, Sven J. van der Lee, Shanthi Mendis, et al., "The Global Impact of Non-communicable Diseases on Healthcare Spending and National Income: A Systematic Review," *European Journal of Epidemiology* 30, no.4 (2015): 251–277.

131. Robert N. Peck, Ethan Green, Jacob Mtabaji, Charles Majinge, Luke R. Smart, Jennifer A. Downs, and Daniel W. Fitzgerald, "Hypertension-Related Diseases as a Common Cause of Hospital Mortality in Tanzania: A 3-Year Prospective Study," *Journal of Hypertension* 31, no. 9 (2013): 1806–1811.

132. John Rose, Thomas G. Weiser, Phil Hider, Leona Wilson, Russel L. Gruen, and Stephen W. Bickler, "Estimated Need for Surgery Worldwide Based on Prevalence of Diseases: A Modeling Strategy for the WHO Global Health Estimate," *Lancet,* Suppl. 2, no. 3 (2015): S13–S20; John Rose, David C. Chang, Thomas G. Weiser, Nicholas J. Kassebaum, and Stephen W. Bickler, "The Role of Surgery in Global Health: Analysis of United States Inpatient Procedure Frequency by Condition Using the Global Burden of Disease 2010 Framework," *PLOS ONE* 9, no. 2 (2014): e89693.

133. Bollyky et al., "Lower-Income Countries That Face the Most Rapid Shift."

134. Joseph L. Dieleman, Gavin Yamey, Elizabeth K. Johnson, Casey M. Graves, Annie Haakenstad, and John G. Meara, "Tracking Global Expenditures on Surgery: Gaps in Knowledge Hinder Progress," *Lancet Global Health* 3 (2015): S2–S4.

135. Institute for Health Metrics and Evaluation, *Financing Global Health 2015.*

136. Andrew Jacobs and Matt Richtel, "How Big Business Got Brazil Hooked on Junk Food," *New York Times*, Sept. 16, 2017; Thomas Reardon, C. Peter Timmer, and Bart Minten, "The Supermarket Revolution in Asia and Emerging Development Strategies to Include Small Farmers," *Proceedings of the National Academy of Sciences* 109, no. 31 (March 10, 2010): 12332–12337; Barry M. Popkin, Linda S. Adair, and Shu Wen Ng, "Now and Then: The Global Nutrition Transition: The Pandemic of Obesity in Developing Countries," *Nutrition Reviews* 70, no. 1 (Jan. 2012): 3–21; David Weatherspoon and Thomas Reardon, "The Rise of Supermarkets in Africa: Implications for Agrifood Systems and the Rural Poor," *Development Policy Review* 21, no. 3 (May 2003): 333–355.

137. Colin K. Khoury, Anne D. Bjorkman, Hannes Dempewolf, Julian Ramirez-Villegas, Luigi Guarino, Andy Jarvis, et al., "Increasing Homogeneity in Global Food Supplies and the Implications for Food Security," *Proceedings of the National Academy of Sciences* 111, no. 11 (2014): 4001–4006.

138. Katharine M. Esson and Stephen R. Leeder, *The Millennium Development Goals and Tobacco Control* (Geneva: World Health Organization, 2004), xi.

139. Thomas J. Bollyky, "Developing Symptoms: Noncommunicable Diseases Go Global," *Foreign Affairs* 91, no. 3 (2012): 136–137.

140. See, e.g., Duff Wilson, "Tobacco Funds Shrink as Obesity Fight Intensifies," *New York Times*, July 27, 2010, http://www.nytimes.com/2010/07/28/health/policy /28obesity.html; Thomas J. Bollyky, *Beyond Ratification: The Future of U.S. Engagement on International Tobacco Control* (Washington, DC: Center for Strategic and International Studies, 2010), 12–13, http://csis.org/files/publication/111210_Bollyky_Bynd Ratifica_WEB.pdf.

141. International Centre for Trade and Sustainable Development, "Tobacco Company Files Claim against Uruguay over Labeling Laws," *Bridges* 14, http://ictsd.org /i/news/bridgesweekly/71988/; Sabrina Tavernise, "Tobacco Firms' Strategy Limits Poorer Nations' Smoking Laws," *New York Times*, Dec. 13, 2013, http://www.nytimes .com/2013/12/13/health/tobacco-industry-tactics-limit-poorer-nations-smoking -laws.html; Thomas J. Bollyky, "The Tobacco Problem in U.S. Trade," *Council on Foreign Relations*, http://www.cfr.org/trade/tobacco-problem-us-trade/p31346.

142. Packard, *History of Global Health*.

143. Centers for Disease Control and Prevention, "Outbreaks Chronology: Ebola Virus Disease," https://www.cdc.gov/vhf/ebola/outbreaks/history/chronology.html.

144. Ian Goldin and Chris Kutarna, *Age of Discovery* (New York: St. Martin's Press, 2016), 182.

145. World Health Organization, "Ebola Situation Report—30 March 2016," March 30, 2016, http://apps.who.int/ebola/current-situation/ebola-situation-report-30 -march-2016; World Health Organization, "Statement on the 9th Meeting of the IHR Emergency Committee Regarding the Ebola Outbreak in West Africa," March 29, 2016, http://www.who.int/mediacentre/news/statements/2016/end-of-ebola -pheic/en/.

146. "Lessons from Polio to Ebola," Editorial, *Lancet Infectious Diseases* 15, no. 8 (2015): 863; Faisal Shuaib, Rajni Gunnala, Emmanuel O. Musa, Frank J. Mahoney, Olukayode Oguntimehin, and Patrick M. Nguku, "Ebola Virus Disease Outbreak— Nigeria, July–September 2014," *Morbidity and Mortality Weekly Report* 63, no. 39 (2014): 867–872.

147. Michiel Hofman and Sokhieng Au, "Introduction" to *The Politics of Fear: Médecins Sans Frontières and the West African Ebola Epidemic*, ed. Michiel Hofman and Sokhieng Au (New York: Oxford University Press, 2017), xvi; Mark Anderson, "Ebola: Airlines Cancel More Flights to Affected Countries," *Guardian*, Aug. 22, 2014.

148. Mark Roland Thomas, Gregory Smith, Francisco H. G. Ferreira, David Evans, Maryla Maliszewska, Marcio Cruz, et al., "The Economic Impact of Ebola on Sub-Saharan Africa: Updated Estimates for 2015," World Bank, January 20, 2015.

149. "The Unfinished Health Agenda in Sub-Saharan Africa," prepared statement by Thomas J. Bollyky, Senior Fellow for Global Health, Economics, and Development Council on Foreign Relations, Before the Senate Foreign Relations Subcommittee on Africa and Global Health Policy, United States Senate First Session, 114th Congress (March 19, 2015); Tong Wu, Charles Perrings, Ann Kinzig, James P. Collins, Ben A. Minteer, Peter Daszak, "Economic Growth, Urbanization, Globalization, and the Risks of Emerging Infectious Diseases in China: A Review," *Ambio* 46 (2017): 18–29.

150. Marco Schäferhoff, Sara Fewer, Jessica Kraus, Emil Richter, Lawrence H. Summers, Jesper Sundewall, et al., "How Much Donor Financing for Health Is Channeled to Global versus Country-Specific Aid Functions?" *Lancet* 286, no. 10011 (2015): 2436–2441; World Health Organization, A66/7, *Proposed Programme Budget 2014–2015*, Sixty-sixth World Health Assembly, April 19, 2013, http://www.who.int/about/resources_planning/A66_7-en.pdf.

151. National Academies of Sciences, Engineering, and Medicine, Health and Medicine Division, Board on Global Health, Committee on Global Health and the Future of the United States, *Global Health and the Future Role of the United States* (Washington, DC: National Academies Press, 2017), 60.

152. Save the Children, "A Wake Up Call: Lessons from Ebola for the World Health Systems," https://www.savethechildren.net/resources; UNICEF, "Under-five and Infant Mortality Rates and Number of Deaths," Oct. 2016, data.unicef.org/topic/child-survival/under-five-mortality.

153. The World Bank, "World Development Indicators," http://data.worldbank.org/data-catalog/world-development-indicators.

154. Sheri Fink, "W.H.O. Members Endorse Resolution to Improve Response to Health Emergencies," *New York Times*, Jan. 26, 2015, https://www.nytimes.com/2015/01/26/world/who-members-endorse-resolution-to-improve-response-to-health-emergencies.html.

155. World Health Organization, "Extended List of Ebola Reviews" (as of May 2016), http://www.who.int/about/evaluation/extended-list-of-ebola-reviews-may2016.pdf?ua=1; Suerie Moon, Jennifer Leigh, Liana Woskie, Francesco Checchi, Victor Dzau, Mosoka Fallah, et al., "Post-Ebola Reforms: Ample Analysis, Inadequate Action," *British Medical Journal* 356 (2017): j280.

156. Coalition for Epidemic Preparedness Innovations, http://cepi.net/.

157. World Bank, International Working Group on Financing Preparedness, *From Panic and Neglect to Investing in Health Security: Financing Pandemic Preparedness at a National Level* (Washington, DC, 2017), 19–24; Gavin Yamey, Marco Schäferhoff, Ole Kristian

Aars, Barry Bloom, Dennis Carroll, Mukesh Chawla, et al., "Financing of International Collective Action for Epidemic and Pandemic Preparedness," *Lancet Global Health* 5 (2017): e742–e743; Josh Michaud, Kellie Moss, and Jennifer Kates, *The U.S. Government and Global Health Security*, The Henry J. Kaiser Family Foundation, Nov. 1, 2017.

158. Lawrence O. Gostin and James G. Hodge Jr., "Zika Virus and Global Health Security," *Lancet Infectious Diseases* 16, no.10 (2016): 1099–1100.

159. Lena H. Sun, "World Leaders Rehearse for a Pandemic That Will Come 'Sooner Than We Expect,'" *Washington Post*, Oct. 24, 2017.

160. William Easterly, *White Man's Burden: Why the West's Efforts to Aid the Rest Have Done So Much Ill and So Little Good* (New York: Penguin, 2007).

161. Dambisa Moyo, *Dead Aid: Why Aid Is Not Working and How There Is a Better Way for Africa* (New York: Allen Lane, 2010); Deaton, *Great Escape*; William Easterly, *Tyranny of Experts: Economists, Dictators, and the Forgotten Rights of the Poor* (New York: Basic Books, 2014).

162. Haidong Wang, Chelsea A Liddell, Matthew M Coates, Meghan D Mooney, Carly E Levitz, Austin E Schumacher, et al., "Global, Regional, National, and Selected Subnational Levels of Stillbirths, Neonatal, Infant, and Under-5 Mortality, 1980–2015: A Systematic Analysis for the Global Burden of Disease Study 2015," *Lancet* 388 (2016): 1725–1774, 1754–1758; David Bishai, Robert Cohen, Y. Natalia Alfonso, Taghreed Adam, Shyama Kuruvilla, Julian Schweitzer, et al., "Factors Contributing to Child Mortality Reductions in 142 Low- and Middle-Income Countries between 1990 and 2010," paper presented at Population Association of America, Annual Meeting, Boston (2014); Matt Andrews, Lant Pritchett, and Michael Woolcock, *Building State Capability: Evidence, Analysis, Action* (Oxford: Oxford University Press, 2017), 14–27.

163. Downie, "Sustaining Improvements to Public Health," 22; Stephen Morrison and Suzanne Brundage, "Advancing Health in Ethiopia: With Fewer Resources, An Uncertain GHI Strategy, and Vulnerabilities on the Ground," Center for Strategic and International Studies, June 2012, 11, https://www.csis.org/analysis/advancing -health-ethiopia.

164. Development Assistance Group, Ethiopia, "ODA to Ethiopia," http://dagethiopia .org/new/oda-to-ethiopia; Janet Fleischman and Katherine Peck, "Imperiling Progress: How Ethiopia's Response to Political Unrest Could Undermine Its Health Gains," Center for Strategic and International Studies, Nov. 3, 2016, https://www.csis.org/ analysis/imperiling-progress.

165. Hailom Banteyerga, Aklilu Kidanu, Lesong Conteh, and Martin McKee, "Ethiopia: Placing Health at the Center of Development," in *"Good Health at Low Cost" 25 Years On: What Makes a Successful Health System?*, ed. Hailom Banteyerga, Martin McKee, and Anne Mills (London: The London School of Hygiene and Tropical Medicine, 2011), 104.

166. Downie, "Sustaining Improvements to Public Health," 10.

167. Banteyerga et al., "Ethiopia," 104.

168. Downie, "Sustaining Improvements to Public Health," 14.

169. Human Rights Watch, "Development without Freedom: How Aid Underwrites Repression in Ethiopia," Oct. 2010, https://www.hrw.org/sites/default/files/reports/ethiopia1010webwcover.pdf.

170. Donald G. McNeil Jr. and Nick Cumming-Bruce, "W.H.O. Elects Ethiopia's Tedros as First Director General from Africa," *New York Times*, May 24, 2017, A6.

171. Wang et al., "Global, Regional, and National Under-5 Mortality." See also Helen Epstein, "Are Tyrants Good for Your Health?" *Lancet* 383 (2014): 1453–1454; Angus Deaton, "Reply to Dr. Agnes Binagwaho," *Boston Review*, July 16, 2015, http://bostonreview.net/blog/angus-deaton-reply-dr-agnes-binagwaho.

172. Lionel Barber, "Women's Rights, Cricket Unites, and an Audience with Paul Kagame: Lionel Barber's Rwanda Diary," *Financial Times*, Aug. 27, 2017.

173. George Rosen, "Political Order and Human Health in Jeffersonian Thought," *Bulletin of the History of Medicine* 26 (1952): 32–44; Porter, *Health, Civilization, and the State*, 57.

174. Amartya Sen, *Development as Freedom* (New York: Anchor Books, 1999), 11.

175. James W. McGuire, *Wealth, Health, and Democracy in East Asia and Latin America* (Cambridge: Cambridge University Press, 2010); Simon Wigley and Arzu Akkoyunlu-Wigley, "The Impact of Democracy and Media Freedom on Under-5 Mortality, 1961–2011," *Social Science and Medicine* 190 (2017): 237–224; Andrew C. Patterson, "Not All Built the Same? A Comparative Study of Electoral Systems and Population Health," *Health and Place* 47 (2017): 90–99; Masayuki Kudamatsu, "Has Democratization Reduced Infant Mortality in Sub-Saharan Africa? Evidence from Micro Data," *Journal of the European Economic Association* 10 (2012): 1294–1317; Timothy J. Besley and Masayuki Kudamatsu, "Health and Democracy," *American Economic Review* 96 (2006): 313–318.

176. Pan American Health Organization, *Core Indicators 2016. Health Situation in the Americas* (PAHO: Washington, DC, 2016), http://iris.paho.org/xmlui/handle/123456789/31289; Timothy J. Besley and Masayuki Kudamatsu, "Making Autocracy Work," LSE STICERD Research Paper No. DEDPS48, April 30, 2008, https://papers.ssrn.com/sol3/papers.cfm?abstract_id=1127017.

177. Angus S. Deaton and Robert Tortora, "People in Sub-Saharan Africa Rate Their Health and Health Care among the Lowest in the World," *Health Affairs* 34, no. 3 (March 2015): 519–527.

Chapter 3: Diseases of Childhood

1. Diary of Ephraim Harris, cited in John Duffy, *Epidemics in Colonial America* (Baton Rouge: Louisiana State University Press, 1953), 174–174.

2. This quote appeared in a 1988 pamphlet published by Sandwell Health Authority in the UK; see "Roald Dahl on Olivia, Writing in 1986," http://roalddahl.com/roald-dahl/timeline/1960s/november-1962.

3. Yuki Furuse, Akira Suzuki, and Hitoshi Oshitani, "Origin of Measles Virus: Divergence from Rinderpest Virus between the 11th and 12th Centuries," *Virology Journal* 7 (2010): 52.

4. Stanford T. Shulman, "The History of Pediatric Infectious Disease," *Pediatric Research* 55 (2004): 163–176.

5. Shulman, "History of Pediatric Infectious Disease."

6. Samuel Preston and Michael R. Haines, *Fatal Years* (Princeton, NJ: Princeton University Press, 1996), 4–6.

7. Mark Woolhouse, Fiona Scott, Zoe Hudson, Richard Howey, and Margo Chase-Topping, "Human Viruses: Discovery and Emergence," *Philosophical Transactions of the Royal Society of London B: Biological Sciences* 367, no. 1604 (2012): 2864–2871.

8. Centers for Disease Control and Prevention, "History of Measles," https://www.cdc.gov/measles/about/history.html; Minal K. Patel, Marta Gacic-Dobo, Peter M. Strebel, Alya Dabbagh, Mick N. Mulders, Jean-Marie Okwo-Bele, et al., "Progress toward Regional Measles Elimination—Worldwide, 2000–2015," *Morbidity Mortality Weekly Report* 65, no. 44 (2016): 1228–1233.

9. Alexander D. Langmuir, "Medical Importance of Measles," *American Journal of Diseases of Children* 103, no. 3 (1962): 224–226. There were significant declines in measles mortality in the United States before the discovery of a vaccine, most likely due to the reduction in secondary infections from antibiotics and improvements in sanitation and nutrition and better public health education. Walter A. Orenstein, Mark J. Papania, and Melinda E. Wharton, "Measles Elimination in the United States," *Journal of Infectious Diseases* 189, suppl. 1 (2004): S1–S3.

10. The Editors of the *Lancet*, "Retraction: Ileal Lymphoid Nodular Hyperplasia, Non-Specific Colitis, and Pervasive Developmental Disorder in Children," *Lancet* 375, no. 9713 (2010): 445.

11. Institute of Medicine, *Adverse Effects of Vaccines: Evidence and Causality* (Washington, DC: The National Academies Press, 2012), https://www.nap.edu/catalog/13164/adverse-effects-of-vaccines-evidence-and-causality; General Medical Council, "Fitness to Practice Panel Hearing," Jan. 28, 2010, http://www.casewatch.org

/foreign/wakefield/gmc_findings.pdf; Clare Dyer, "Wakefield Was Dishonest and Irresponsible Over MMR Research, Says GMC," *British Medical Journal* 340 (2010).

12. Centers for Disease Control and Prevention, "Measles Cases and Outbreaks," https://www.cdc.gov/measles/cases-outbreaks.html.

13. Brian Greenwood, "The Contribution of Vaccination to Global Health: Past, Present and Future," *Philosophical Transactions of the Royal Society of London B: Biological Sciences* 369, no. 1645 (2014), doi:10.1098/rstb.2013.0433.

14. Lawrence K. Altman, "How Tiny Errors in Africa Led to a Global Triumph," *New York Times*, Sept. 26, 2011, http://www.nytimes.com/2011/09/27/health/27docs.html.

15. Randall M. Packard, *History of Global Health* (Baltimore: Johns Hopkins University Press, 2016), 256.

16. Adam Fifield, *A Mighty Purpose: How Jim Grant Sold the World on Saving Its Children* (New York: Other Press, 2016), 5–6.

17. Fifield, *Mighty Purpose*, 52; Packard, *History of Global Health*, 256–257.

18. Packard, *History of Global Health*, 258, 265.

19. Fifield, *Mighty Purpose*, 126, 143–169, 183.

20. Fifield, *Mighty Purpose*, 120–121.

21. Peter Adamson, Carol Bellamy, Kul Gautam, Richard Jolly, Nyi Nyi, Mary Racelis, et al., *Jim Grant: UNICEF Visionary*, ed. Richard Jolly (Florence: UNICEF Innocenti Research Centre, 2001), 59.

22. Bill Gates, "Jim Grant's Child Survival Revolution," *Impatient Optimists* (blog), Bill and Melinda Gates Foundation, Feb. 17, 2011, http://www.impatientoptimists .org/Posts/2011/02/Jim-Grants-Child-Survival-Revolution.

23. Packard, *History of Global Health*, 216.

24. William Foege, "The Power of Immunization," in *The Progress of Nations* (New York: UNICEF, 2000).

25. Gavi, "Annual Contributions and Proceeds," Sept. 30, 2016, http://www.gavi .org/funding/donor-contributions-pledges/annual-contributions-and-proceeds/.

26. World Health Organization, "Global and Regional Immunization Profile 2016" (data received as of July 19, 2017), http://www.who.int/immunization/monitoring _surveillance/data/gs_gloprofile.pdf?ua=1.

27. Patel et al., "Progress toward Regional Measles Elimination," 1228–1233.

28. World Bank DataBank, "GDP Per Capita (Current US$)," http://data.worldbank .org/indicator/NY.GDP.PCAP.CD?end=2015&start=1976.

29. Yang Jisheng, *Tombstone: The Great Chinese Famine, 1958–1962* (New York: Farrar, Straus and Giroux, 2013), 28.

30. Steven Radelet, *The Great Surge: The Ascent of the Developing World* (New York: Simon and Schuster, 2015), 36; Nancy Birdsall, "Middle Class Heroes," *Foreign Affairs*, March–April 2016, https://www.foreignaffairs.com/articles/2016-02-15/middle-class-heroes.

31. World Bank DataBank, "Life Expectancy at Birth, Total (Years)," http://data.worldbank.org/indicator/SP.DYN.LE00.IN?end=2014&start=1960.

32. James C. Riley, *Low-Income, Social Growth, and Good Health: A History of Twelve Countries* (Berkeley: University of California Press/Milbank Books on Health and the Public, 2007), 111.

33. Riley, *Low-Income, Social Growth*, 111.

34. Riley, *Low-Income, Social Growth*, 110–111; David Hipgrave, "Communicable Disease Control in China: From Mao to Now," *Journal of Global Health* 1, no. 2 (2011): 224–238.

35. Xiaoping Fang, *Barefoot Doctors and Western Medicine in China* (Rochester, NY: University of Rochester Press, 2012), 25–28; Riley, *Low-Income, Social Growth*, 25–28, 112; Tina Phillips Johnson and Yi-Li Wu, "Maternal and Child Health in Nineteenth- to Twenty-First-Century China," in *Medical Transitions in Twentieth-Century China*, ed. Bridie J. Andrews and Mary Brown Bullock (Bloomington: Indiana University Press, 2014), 61–64.

36. Miriam Gross, *Farewell to the God of Plague: Chairman Mao's Campaign to Deworm China* (Oakland, CA: Berkeley Press, 2016), 1–2, 7, 18, 20.

37. Kerrie L. MacPherson, "Hong Kong and China and the Double Disease Burden," in *Health Transitions and the Double Disease Burden in Asia and the Pacific*, ed. Milton J. Lewis and Kerrie L. MacPherson (New York: Routledge, 2013), 60.

38. Hipgrave, "Communicable Disease Control in China," 226; Xingjian Xu, "Control of Communicable Diseases in the People's Republic of China," *Asia Pacific Journal of Public Health* 7, no. 2 (1994): 123–131.

39. Robert William Fogel, "New Findings on Secular Trends in Nutrition and Mortality: Some Implications for Population Theory," in *Handbook of Population and Family Economics*, vol. 1A, ed. Mark R. Rosenzweig and Oded Stark (Boston: Elsevier, 1997), 433–481.

40. Hoyt Bleakley, "Disease and Development: Evidence from Hookworm Eradication in the American South," *Quarterly Journal of Economics* 122, no. 1 (2007): 73–117; Jere R. Behrman and Mark R. Rosenzweig, "Returns to Birthweight," *Review of Economics and Statistics* 86, no. 2 (2004): 586–601.

41. Dean T. Jamison, Lawrence H. Summers, George Alleyne, Kenneth J. Arrow, Seth Berkley, Agnes Binagwaho, et al., "Global Health 2035: A World Converging within a Generation," *Lancet* 383, no. 9908 (2013): 1898–1955.

42. Universal Health Coverage Coalition, "Economists' Declaration," http://universal healthcoverageday.org/economists-declaration/.

43. Daron Acemoglu and Simon Johnson, "Disease and Development: The Effect of Life Expectancy on Economic Growth," *Journal of Political Economy* 115, no. 6 (2007): 925–985.

44. Quamrul H. Ashraf, Ashley Lester, and David N. Weil, "When Does Improving Health Raise GDP?" (working paper, The National Bureau of Economic Research, no. 14449, 2008), 26.

45. Susan Greenhalgh and Edwin A. Winkler, *Governing China's Population: From Leninist to Neoliberal Biopolitics* (Palo Alto, CA: Stanford University Press, 2005), 17, 55–92; Tyrene White, *China's Longest Campaign: Birth Planning in the People's Republic, 1949–2005* (Ithaca: Cornell University Press, 2006), 19–41; Johnson and Wu, "Maternal and Child Health," 61–64; Riley, *Low-Income, Social Growth*, 113; Joe Studwell, *How Asia Works: Success and Failure in the World's Most Dynamic Region* (London: Profile Books, 2013), xxii, 21–22.

46. Deaton, *Great Escape*, 38–39.

47. David E. Bloom, David Canning, and Jocelyn E. Finlay, "Population Aging and Economic Growth in Asia," in *The Economic Consequences of Demographic Change in East Asia*, NBER-EASE vol. 19, ed. Takatoshi Ito and Andrew Rose (Chicago: University of Chicago Press, 2010), 61–89.

48. Paul Krugman, "The Myth of Asia's Miracle," *Foreign Affairs*, Nov.–Dec. 1994, 73.

49. Robert J. Gordon, *The Rise and Fall of American Growth* (Princeton, NJ: Princeton University Press, 2016), 209.

50. Ruchir Sharma, "The Demographics of Stagnation: Why People Matter for Economic Growth," *Foreign Affairs*, March–April 2016, https://www.foreignaffairs.com /articles/world/2016-02-15/demographics-stagnation. Economists have also partially attributed past episodes of spectacular economic growth, such as in nineteenth-century British industrial cities, to young adults representing a disproportionately large share of the population. Jeffrey G. Williamson, *Coping with City Growth during the British Industrial Revolution* (Cambridge: Cambridge University Press, 2002), 30–31.

51. Andrew Mason, "Demographic Transition and Demographic Dividends in Developed and Developing Countries" (submitted paper, *Proceedings of the United Nations Expert Group Meeting on Social and Economic Implications of Changing Population Age Structures*, Mexico City, Aug. 31, 2005), http://www.un.org/esa/population /meetings/Proceedings_EGM_Mex_2005/mason.pdf.

52. David S. Canning, Sangeeta Raja, and Abdo S. Yazbeck, eds., *Africa's Demographic Transition: Dividend or Disaster?* (Washington, DC: World Bank, 2015), 50.

53. Mark R. Montgomery and Barney Cohen, eds., *From Death to Birth: Mortality Decline and Reproductive Change* (Washington, DC: The National Academies Press, 1998), 74–111; see also Bill Gates and Melinda Gates, "Annual Letter 2014," Bill and Melinda Gates Foundation, http://www.gatesfoundation.org/Who-We-Are/Resources -and-Media/Annual-Letters-List/Annual-Letter-2014.

54. Canning, Raja, and Yazbeck, *Africa's Demographic Transition*, 26.

55. Jere R. Behrman and Hans-Peter Kohler, "Quantity, Quality, and Mobility of Population," in *Toward a Better Global Economy: Policy Implications for Citizens Worldwide in the 21st Century*, ed. Franklin Allen et al. (Oxford: Oxford University Press, 2014), 141; Daron Acemoglu and James Robinson, *Why Nations Fail: The Origins of Power, Prosperity, and Poverty* (New York: Crown, 2012), 431.

56. Studwell, *How Asia Works*, 13–15.

57. Studwell, *How Asia Works*, 223.

58. Tyler Cowen, "Economic Development in an 'Average Is Over' World" (working paper, 2016).

59. Richard Baldwin, "Trade and Industrialisation after Globalisation's 2nd Unbundling: How Building and Joining a Supply Chain Are Different and Why It Matters," NBER Working Paper No. 17716, 2011.

60. Thomas J. Bollyky and Petros C. Mavroidis, "Trade, Social Preferences and Regulatory Cooperation: The New WTO-Think," *Journal of International Economic Law* 20, no. 1 (2017): 1–30.

61. Marcos Cueto, *The Value of Health: A History of the Pan American Health Organization* (Washington, DC: Boydell & Brewer, 2007), 107–125.

62. Albert Esteve, Joan Garcia-Roman, Ron Lesthaeghe, and Antonio Lopez-Gay, "The 'Second Demographic Transition' Features in Latin America: The 2010 Update" (unpublished manuscript, Centre d'Estudis Demografics, Universitat Autonoma de Barcelona, Barcelona, 2012), http://www.vub.ac.be/demography/wp-content /uploads/2016/02/LatAm_SDT_update.doc.

63. Canning, Raja, and Yazbeck, *Africa's Demographic Transition*, 50; Jeffrey G. Williamson, "Latin American Inequality: Colonial Origins, Commodity Booms, or a Missed 20th Century Leveling?" NBER Working Paper No. 20915, 2015.

64. Mason, "Demographic Transition."

65. Institute for Health Metrics and Evaluation, Country Profiles, "Kenya," http:// www.healthdata.org/kenya.

66. Jeffrey Gettleman, "36 Hours in Nairobi, Kenya," *New York Times*, Dec. 15, 2016, https://www.nytimes.com/interactive/2016/12/15/travel/what-to-do-36-hours-in-nairobi-kenya.html.

67. Eric Kramon and Daniel N. Posner, "Kenya's New Constitution," *Journal of Democracy* 22, no. 2 (2011): 89–103.

68. Steve Johnson, "Kenya a Rare Bright Spot in Emerging Markets Gloom," *Financial Times*, Feb. 4, 2016, https://www.ft.com/content/ffb0470c-c9cd-11e5-a8ef-ea66e967dd44.

69. World Bank, *Kenya Economic Update* (Washington, DC: World Bank Group, June 10, 2014), 6, 12–13.

70. World Bank, *Kenya Economic Update*, 35.

71. World Bank, *Kenya Economic Update*, 5–6, 23.

72. Rakesh Kochhar, "A Global Middle Class Is More Promise Than Reality: From 2001 to 2011, Nearly 700 Million Step Out of Poverty, but Most Only Barely," *Pew Research Center*, July 8, 2015, http://www.pewglobal.org/2015/07/08/a-global-middle-class-is-more-promise-than-reality/.

73. Eliya M. Zulu, Donatien Beguy, Alex C. Ezeh, Philippe Bocquier, Nyovani J. Madise, John Cleland, and Jane Falkingham, "Overview of Migration, Poverty and Health Dynamics in Nairobi City's Slum Settlements," *Journal of Urban Health* 88, supplement 2 (2011): S185–S199; Demographia, *Demographia World Urban Areas*, 12th annual ed. (Belleville, IL: Demographia, April 2016).

74. Zulu et al., "Overview of Migration, Poverty and Health Dynamics," S186.

75. UN-Habitat, *The State of African Cities 2010: Governance, Inequalities and Urban Land Markets* (Nairobi, Kenya: UN-Habitat, 2010), 29.

76. World Bank, *Kenya Economic Update*, 35.

77. Joseph L. Dieleman, Tara Templin, Nafis Sadat, Patrick Reidy, Abigail Chapin, Kyle Foreman, et al., "National Spending on Health by Source for 184 Countries between 2013 and 2040," *Lancet* 387 (2016): 2521–2535.

78. World Bank, *Kenya Economic Update*, 34.

79. Colin H. Kahl, *States, Scarcity, and Civil Strife in the Developing World* (Princeton, NJ: Princeton University Press, 2006), 117.

80. Jeffrey Gettleman, "Kenya's Collective 'Uh-Oh': Another Election Is Coming," *New York Times*, June 6, 2016, A4; Nela Wadekar, "Kenyan Democracy's Missed Opportunity," *New Yorker*, Aug. 16, 2017.

81. Helen Epstein, "Kenya: The Election and the Cover-Up," *New York Review of Books*, Aug. 30, 2017.

82. "Kenya Watchdog Says 92 People Killed in Election Violence," *Associated Press*, Dec. 20, 2017; Humphrey Malalo, "University of Nairobi Closed as Anger Rises Over Police Brutality," *Reuters*, Oct. 3, 2017; John Campbell, "Low Turnout, Protests, and No End in Sight for Kenyan Election Crisis," *CFR.org*, Oct. 25, 2017.

83. Kimiko de Freytas-Tamura, "Kenya Court Says It Nullified Election Over Possible Hacking," *New York Times*, Sept. 20, 2017.

84. "Kenya's Giant Step for Fair Elections," *New York Times*, Sept. 3, 2017; John Campbell, "Uneasy Stalemate in Post-Election Kenya," *CFR.org*, Aug. 21, 2017.

85. Robert Barro and Jong-Wha Lee, "A New Data Set of Educational Attainment in the World, 1950–2010," *Journal of Development Economics* 104 (2013): 184–198.

86. Michael A. Clemens and David McKenzie, "Why Don't Remittances Appear to Affect Growth?" World Bank Policy Research Working Paper No. 6856, 2014. See World Bank Development Indicators, "Foreign direct investment, net inflows (BoP, current US$)"; "Personal remittances, received (current US$)"; "Net official development assistance and official aid received (current US$)" (last visited Dec. 22, 2017), https://data.worldbank.org/indicator/BX.KLT.DINV.CD.WD; https://data.worldbank .org/indicator/BX.TRF.PWKR.CD.DT; https://data.worldbank.org/indicator/DT.ODA .ALLD.CD.

87. African Development Bank, *African Economic Outlook 2017: Entrepreneurship and Industrialization* (Abidjan: African Development Group, 2017), 5.

88. African Development Bank, *Annual Effectiveness Review 2016: Accelerating the Pace of Change* (Abidjan: African Development Group, 2016), 38–39.

89. Ejaz Ghani and Stephen D. O'Connell, "Can Service Be a Growth Escalator in Low-Income Countries?" World Bank Policy Research Working Paper No. 6971, July 2014, 14.

90. Cowen, "Economic Development," 4–5.

91. Cowen, "Economic Development," 5.

92. Dani Rodrik, "Premature Deindustrialization," *Journal of Economic Growth* 21 (2016): 1.

93. Marcel P. Timmer, Gaaitzen de Vries and Klaas de Vries, "Patterns of Structural Change in Developing Countries," Groningen Growth and Development Centre Working Paper No. 149 (July 2014), http://www.ggdc.net/publications/memoran dum/gd149.pdf.

94. Deon Filmer and Louise Fox, *Youth Employment in Sub-Saharan Africa* (Washington, DC: World Bank, 2014), 30–35.

95. Dani Rodrik, "Past, Present, and Future of Economic Growth," *Challenge* 57, no. 3 (2014): 5–39.

96. Janet Ceglowski, Stephen Golub, Aly Mbaye, and Varun Prasad, "Can Africa Compete with China in Manufacturing? The Role of Relative Unit Labor Costs," manuscript, Swarthmore College, 2015; Alan Gelb, Christian J. Meyer, Vijaya Ramachandran, and Divyanshi Wadhwa, "Can Africa Be a Manufacturing Destination? Labor Costs in Comparative Perspective," Center for Global Development Working Paper 466 (2017).

97. World Bank, *World Development Report 2016: Digital Dividends* (Washington, DC: World Bank, 2016), 22.

98. World Bank, *World Development Report 2016*, 22–23.

99. Howard L. Sirkin, Justin Rose, and Michael Zinzer, *The US Manufacturing Renaissance: How Shifting Global Economics are Creating an American Comeback* (Boston: Boston Consulting Group, 2012), http://kw.wharton.upenn.edu/made-in-america-again/.

100. Kevin Sneader and Jonathan Woetzel, "China's Impending Robot Revolution," *Wall Street Journal*, Aug. 3, 2016.

101. Cowen, "Economic Development," 10.

102. Marcelo Giugale, "Can Services Drive Africa's Development?" *Huffington Post: The World Post*, Sept. 5, 2016, http://www.huffingtonpost.com/marcelo-giugale/can-services-drive-africa_b_11866756.html; Bineswaree Bolaky, "Unlocking the Potential of Africa's Services for Transformation," *Bridges Africa* 5, no. 4, May 19, 2016.

103. Richard Dobbs, James Manyika, and Jonathan Woetzel, *No Ordinary Disruption: The Four Global Forces Breaking All the Trends* (New York: Public Affairs, 2015), 93–110.

104. Kochhar, "A Global Middle Class Is More Promise," 6.

105. Martha Chen, Sally Roever, and Caroline Skinner, "Editorial: Urban Livelihoods: Reframing Theory and Policy," *Environment and Urbanization* 28, no. 2 (2016): 331–342.

106. Cowen, "Economic Development," 4.

107. Ericcson, *Ericcson Mobility Report* (Stockholm: Ericcson, June 2017), 33–35, https://www.ericsson.com/assets/local/mobility-report/documents/2017/ericsson-mobility-report-june-2017.pdf.

108. Jim Yong Kim, "Rethinking Development Finance" (speech, London, April 11, 2017), The World Bank, http://www.worldbank.org/en/news/speech/2017/04/11/speech-by-world-bank-group-president-jim-yong-kim-rethinking-development-finance.

109. Sanders Korenman and David Neumark, "Cohort Crowding and Youth Labor Markets (A Cross-National Analysis)," in *Youth Employment and Joblessness*

in Advanced Countries, ed. David G. Blachflower and Richard B. Freeman (Chicago: University of Chicago Press, 2000), 57–106.

110. Jennifer Keller and Mustapha K. Nabli, "The Macroeconomics of Labor Market Outcomes in MENA over the 1990s: How Growth Has Failed to Keep Pace with a Burgeoning Labor Market" (working paper, World Bank, Washington DC, June 2002), http://siteresources.worldbank.org/INTMENA/Resources/Labmarkout-comes.pdf.

111. Tarik Yousef, "Youth in the Middle East and North Africa: Demography, Employment, and Conflict," in *Youth Explosion in Developing World Cities: Approaches to Reducing Poverty and Conflict in an Urban Age*, ed. Blair A. Ruble et al. (Washington, DC: Wilson Center, 2003), 12.

112. Yousef, "Youth in the Middle East."

113. Kahl, *States, Scarcity, and Civil Strife*, 35–39.

114. Jack A. Goldstone, "Theory of Political Demography: Human and Institutional Reproduction," in *Political Demography: How Population Changes Are Reshaping International Security and National Politics*, ed. Jack A. Goldstone et al. (Boulder, CO: Paradigm Publishers, 2012), 27.

115. Indermit S. Gill and Homi Kharas, "The Middle-Income Trap Turns Ten," World Bank, working paper, Washington, DC, Aug. 2015), http://documents.worldbank.org/curated/en/291521468179640202/pdf/WPS7403.pdf.

116. African Development Bank, *Annual Effectiveness Review 2016*, 47; Therese F. Azeng and Thierry U. Yogo, "Youth Unemployment and Political Instability in Selected Developing Countries," African Development Bank Working Paper No. 171, May 2013.

Chapter 4: Diseases of Settlement

1. United Nations, Department of Economic and Social Affairs, Population Division, *World Urbanization Prospects: The 2014 Revision, Highlights* (ST/ESA/SER.A/352) (New York: United Nations, 2014), 2.

2. Paul Slack, *The Impact of Plague in Tudor and Stuart England* (London: Routledge and Kegan Paul, 1985), 313–326; Nükhet Varlık, "New Science and Old Sources: Why the Ottoman Experience of Plague Matters," *Medieval Global* 1 (2014): 193–224.

3. Paul M. Hohenberg and Lynn H. Lees, *The Making of Urban Europe, 1000–1994* (Cambridge, MA: Harvard University Press), 7; John Duffy, *The Sanitarians: A History of American Public Health* (Urbana: University of Illinois Press), 37.

4. Szreter, *Health and Wealth: Studies in History and Policy* (Rochester: University of Rochester Press, 2007), 112, 126.

5. Christine L. Corton, *London Fog: The Biography* (Cambridge, MA: Belknap Press of Harvard University Press, 2015), 77–80.

6. Otto Bettman, *The Good Old Days—They Were Terrible!* (New York: Random House, 1974), 2.

7. Martin V. Melosi, *The Sanitary City* (Baltimore: Johns Hopkins University Press, 2000), 26.

8. Melosi, *Sanitary City*, 62.

9. George Rosen, *A History of Public Health* (Baltimore: Johns Hopkins University Press, 1991), 12, 114–115; Great Britain Historical GIS, University of Portsmouth, "Manchester District through time? Population Statistics: Total Population, A Vision of Britain through Time," http://www.visionofbritain.org.uk/unit/10033007/cube /TOT_POP.

10. Angus Deaton, *The Great Escape: Health, Wealth, and the Origins of Inequality* (Princeton, NJ: Princeton University Press, 2013), 94; J. N. Hays, *The Burdens of Disease: Epidemics and Human Response in Western History* (New Brunswick, NJ: Rutgers University Press, 2009), 143.

11. Charles Dickens, "The Trouble Water Question," *Household Words, a Weekly Journal*, April 13, 1850.

12. Duffy, *Sanitarians*, 87.

13. Bettman, *Good Old Days*, 14.

14. Melosi, *Sanitary City*, 179.

15. C. Rosenberg, *The Cholera Years: The United States in 1832, 1849, and 1866* (Chicago: University of Chicago Press, 1962), 17–19.

16. Rosenberg, *Cholera Years*, 88.

17. John Duffy, *A History of Public Health in New York City, 1625–1866* (New York: Russell Sage Foundation, 1968), 151–152; Rosenberg, *Cholera Years*, 19–20.

18. Melosi, *Sanitary City*, 180.

19. Dorothy Porter, *Health, Civilization, and the State: A History of Public Health from Ancient to Modern Times* (New York: Routledge Books, 1999), 97–162.

20. Melosi, *Sanitary City*, 18–23; Louis P. Cain and Elyce J. Rotella, "Death and Spending: Urban Mortality and Municipal Expenditure on Sanitation," *Annales de Démographie Historique* 1 (2001): 139–154.

21. Edward Glaeser, *Triumph of the City: How Our Greatest Invention Makes Us Richer, Smarter, Greener, Healthier, and Happier* (London: Pan Books, 2012), 99; Rosenberg, *Cholera Years*, 19–20; Duffy, *Sanitarians*, 48.

22. Melosi, *Sanitary City*, 17; Christopher Hamlin, *A Science of Impurity: Water Analysis in Nineteenth Century Britain* (Berkeley: University of California Press, 1990), 81.

23. David Cutler and Grant Miller, "The Role of Public Health Improvements in Health Advances: The Twentieth-Century United States," *Demography* 42, no. 1 (2005): 1–22, 3–4.

24. Mark Achtman, "How Old Are Bacterial Pathogens?" *Proceedings of the Royal Society of London B: Biological Sciences* 283 (2016): 20160990; Daniela Brites and Sebastien Gagneux, "Co-evolution of Mycobacterium Tuberculosis and *Homo sapiens*," *Immunological Reviews* 264 (2015): 6–24; Thomas M. Daniel, "The History of Tuberculosis," *Respiratory Medicine* 100, no. 11 (Nov. 2006): 1862–1870, 1863.

25. Daniel, "History of Tuberculosis."

26. F. B. Smith, *The Retreat of Tuberculosis 1850–1950* (New York: Croom Helm, 1988), 1, 18.

27. Helen Bynum, *Spitting Blood: The History of Tuberculosis* (Oxford: Oxford University Press, 2012), 112–113.

28. Bynum, *Spitting Blood*; Zhang Yixia and Mark Elvin, "Environment and Tuberculosis in Modern China," in *Sediments of Time: Environment and Society in Chinese History*, ed. Mark Elvin and Cuirong Liu (Cambridge: Cambridge University Press, 1998), 533–539.

29. *Complete Works of Marx and Engels*, vol. 23 (Beijing: People's Publishing House, 1979), 529.

30. Cormac Ó Gráda, "Cast Back into the Dark Ages of Medicine? The Challenge of Antimicrobial Resistance" (working paper, UCD Center for Economic Research, May 2015), 3.

31. Daniel, "History of Tuberculosis," 1864.

32. C. Tsiamis, E. T. Piperaki, G. Kalantzis, E. Poulakou Rebelakou, N. Tompros, E. Thalassinou, et al., "Lord Byron's Death: A Case of Late Malarial Relapse?" *Le Infezioni in Medicina* 23, no. 3 (2015): 288–295.

33. Hays, *Burdens of Disease*, chap. 8; Mark Harrison, *Disease and the Modern World: 1500 to the Present Day* (Cambridge: Polity Press, 2004), 87.

34. Johnson, *The Ghost Map: The Story of London's Most Terrifying Epidemic—and How It Changed Science, Cities, and the Modern World* (London: Riverhead Books, 2007), 34; John Noble Wilford, "How Epidemics Helped Shape the Modern Metropolis," *New York Times*, April 15, 2008.

35. Christopher Hamlin, *Cholera: The Biography* (New York: Oxford University Press, 2009), 11.

36. Mark D. Hardt, *History of Infectious Diseases in Urban Societies* (London: Lexington Books, 2016), 112–113.

37. Gerry Kearns, "The Urban Penalty and the Population History of England," in *Society, Health and Population During The Demographic Transition*, ed. Anders Brändström and Lars-Göran Tedebrand (Stockholm: Almqvist and Wiksell International, 1988), 213–236.

38. Charles Dickens, "A Winter Vision," *Harper's New Monthly Magazine* 2 (1851): 360.

39. Bairoch, *Cities and Economic Development: From the Dawn of History to the Present* (Chicago: University of Chicago Press, 1988), 206; Kyle Harper, *The Fate of Rome: Climate, Disease, and the End of an Empire* (Princeton, NJ: Princeton University Press, 2017), 72–91.

40. Hohenberg and Lees, *The Making of Urban Europe*, 257–258.

41. David Rosner, "Introduction," in *Hives of Sickness: Public Health and Epidemics in the History of the City of New York*, ed. David Rosner (New York: Museum of the City of New York, 1995), 3.

42. Cutler and Miller, "Role of Public Health Improvements," 1–2.

43. Duffy, *History of Public Health*, 291.

44. Deaton, *Great Escape*, 94–95; Jeffrey G. Williamson, *Coping with City Growth during the British Industrial Revolution* (Cambridge: Cambridge University Press, 1990), 8–52.

45. Joel E. Cohen, "Beyond Population: Everyone Counts in Development" (working paper, Center for Global Development, no. 220, July 26, 2010); Pamela Sharpe, "Explaining the Short Stature of the Poor: Chronic Childhood Disease and Growth in Nineteenth-Century England," *Economic History Review* 65, no. 4 (2012): 1475–1494.

46. Daniel Knutsson, "The Effect of Introducing Clean Piped Water on Mortality in Stockholm: 1850–1872," unpublished paper, Stockholm University, 2016.

47. Richard J. Evans, *Death in Hamburg: Society and Politics in Cholera Years* (London: Penguin, 2005), 197.

48. Michael R. Haines, "The Urban Morality Transition in the United States: 1800–1940," *Annales de Demographie Historique* (2001): 33–64.

49. Edward Meeker, "The Social Rate of Return on Investment in Public Health, 1880–1910," *Journal of Economic History* 34, no. 2 (June 1974): 392–421.

50. Hohenberg and Lees, *Making of Urban Europe*, 258–259; Mark R. Montgomery, Richard Stren, Barney Cohen, and Holly E. Reed, eds., *Cities Transformed: Demographic Change and Its Implications in the Developing World Panel on Urban Population Dynamics* (Oxon: Earthscan, 2003), 271.

51. Kota Ogasawara et al., "Public Health Improvements and Mortality in Early Twentieth-Century Japan," unpublished paper, Tokyo Institute of Technology, 2015.

52. Bynum, *Spitting Blood*, 173.

53. Bynum, *Spitting Blood*, 113; Szreter, *Health and Wealth*, 127.

54. Nancy Tomes, *The Gospel of Germs: Men, Women, and the Microbe in American Life* (Cambridge, MA: Harvard University Press, 1999), 114–121; John Duffy, "Social Impact of Disease in the Late Nineteenth Century," *Bulletin of New York Academy of Medicine* 47, no. 7 (1971): 797–810.

55. Hays, *Burdens of Disease*, 160–161.

56. Szreter, *Health and Wealth*, 119.

57. Szreter, *Health and Wealth*, 220–225; William H. McNeill, *Plagues and Peoples*, 3rd ed. (New York: Anchor Books and Random House, 1998), 276–278.

58. Quoted in Melosi, *Sanitary City*, 53.

59. Lee Jackson, *Dirty Old London: The Victorian Fight against Filth* (New Haven, CT: Yale University Press, 2015), 98–99.

60. Melosi, *Sanitary City*, 53.

61. Hamlin, *Cholera*, 139–141; Robert Buckley, "Financing Sewers in the 19th Century's Largest Cities: A Prequel for African Cities?" George Washington University–World Bank Urban Conference Paper, Sept. 2017 (on file with author).

62. Porter, *Health, Civilization, and the State*, 153; Duffy, *Sanitarians*, 53; Jackson, *Dirty Old London*, 99.

63. Porter, *Health, Civilization, and the State*, 15; Rosenberg, *Cholera Years*, 192–212; Duffy, *Sanitarians*, 120.

64. Porter, *Health, Civilization, and the State*, 153–154; Melosi, *Sanitary City*, 46.

65. Nava Ashraf, Edward L. Glaeser, and Giacomo A. M. Ponzetto, "Infrastructure, Incentives, and Institutions," *American Economic Review: Papers & Proceedings* 106, no. 5 (2016): 77–82.

66. Christopher Hamlin, "Cholera Forcing: The Myth of the Good Epidemic and the Coming of Good Water," *American Journal of Public Health* 99 (2009): 1946–1954.

67. John C. Brown, "Coping with Crisis? The Diffusion of Waterworks in Late Nineteenth-Century German Towns," *Journal of Economic History* 48 (1988): 307–318; Hamlin, "Cholera Forcing."

68. Melosi, *Sanitary City*, 18–19; Hamlin, "Cholera Forcing"; Williamson, *Coping with City Growth*, 284.

69. McNeill, *Plagues and Peoples*, 278.

70. Montgomery et al., *Cities Transformed*, 271.

71. Susan B. Carter, "City Waterworks, by Type of Ownership: 1800–1924," table Dh236–239 in *Historical Statistics of the United States, Earliest Times to the Present*, millennial ed., ed. Susan B. Carter, Scott Sigmund Gartner, Michael R. Haines, Alan L. Olmstead, Richard Sutch, and Gavin Wright (New York: Cambridge University Press, 2006).

72. Robert J. Gordon, *The Rise and Fall of American Growth: The U.S. Standard of Living since the Civil War* (Princeton, NJ: Princeton University Press, 2016), 216.

73. Scott E. Masten, "Public Utility Ownership in 19th-Century America: The 'Aberrant' Case of Water," *Journal of Law, Economics, and Organization* 27, no. 3 (2011): 604–654, 609.

74. David Cutler and Grant Miller, "The Role of Public Health Improvements in Health Advances: The Twentieth-Century United States," *Demography* 42, no. 1 (2005): 1–22.

75. Gordon, *Rise and Fall of American Growth*, 123, 207.

76. Melosi, *Sanitary City*, 35.

77. Robert Millward and Sally Sheard, "The Urban Fiscal Problem, 1870–1914: Government Expenditure and Finance in England and Wales," *Economic History Review* 48 (1995): 501–535; Melosi, *Sanitary City*, 75–77.

78. Brown, "Coping with Crisis?," 307; Millward and Sheard, "The Urban Fiscal Problem"; John B. Legler, Richard Sylla, and John J. Wallis, "U.S. City Finances and the Growth of Government, 1850–1902," *Journal of Economic History* 48 (1988): 347–356; Hamlin, *Cholera*; Buckley, "Financing Sewers in the 19th Century"; Melosi, *Sanitary City*, 120–121.

79. Glaeser, *Triumph of the City*.

80. United Nations, "Growth of the World's Urban and Rural Population, 1920–2000" (New York: United Nations, 1969), table 8.

81. Joshua Nalibow Ruxin, "Magic Bullet: The History of Oral Rehydration Therapy," *Medical History* 38 (1994): 363–397, 380.

82. Public Radio International, "A Simple Solution: The History of ORS in Bangladesh," June 25, 2013, https://www.pri.org/stories/2013-06-25/simple-solution-history-ors-bangladesh.

83. Billy Woodward, *Scientists Greater Than Einstein* (Fresno, CA: Quill Driver Books, 2009), 113.

84. "Control of Diarrhoeal Diseases: WHO's Programme Takes Shape," *WHO Chronicle* 32, no. 10 (1978): 369.

85. A. Mushtaque R. Chowdhury, Abbas Bhuiya, Mahbub Elahi Chowdhury, Sabrina Rasheed, Zakir Hussain, and Lincoln C. Chen, "The Bangladesh Paradox: Exceptional Health Achievement Despite Economic Poverty," *Lancet* 382, no. 9906 (2013): 1734–1745, 1739.

86. Woodward, *Scientists Greater Than Einstein*, 135; Amy Yee, "In Bangladesh, a Half-Century of Saving Lives with Data," *New York Times*, Nov. 17, 2015, https://opinionator.blogs.nytimes.com/2015/11/17/in-bangladesh-a-half-century-of-saving-lives-with-data/?_r=0.

87. Ruxin, "Magic Bullet," 389.

88. Atul Gawande, "Slow Ideas," *New Yorker*, July 20, 2013, http://www.newyorker.com/magazine/2013/07/29/slow-ideas; Ruxin, "Magic Bullet," 389.

89. Naomi Hossain, *The Aid Lab: Understanding Bangladesh's Unexpected Success* (Oxford: Oxford University Press, 2017), 3–6, 91–141.

90. Gawande, "Slow Ideas."

91. Tracey Pérez Koehlmoos, Ziaul Islam, Shahela Anwar, Shaikh A. Shahed Hossain, Rukhsana Gazi, Peter Kim Streatfield, and Abbas Uddin Bhuiya, "Health Transcends Poverty: The Bangladesh Experience," in *"Good Health at Low Cost" 25 Years on: What Makes a Successful Health System?* (London: London School of Hygiene and Tropical Medicine, 2011).

92. Amy Yee, "The Power, and Process, of a Simple Solution," *New York Times*, Aug. 14, 2014, https://opinionator.blogs.nytimes.com/2014/08/14/the-power-and-process-of-a-simple-solution/.

93. Olivier Fontaine, Paul Garner, and M. K. Bhan, "Oral Rehydration Therapy: The Simple Solution for Saving Lives," *British Medical Journal* 334 (2007): s14.

94. Gawande, "Slow Ideas."

95. "Water with Sugar and Salt," *Lancet* 312, no. 8084 (1978): 300.

96. Chowdhury et al., "Bangladesh Paradox," 1739; Fahima Chowdhury, Mohammad Arif Rahman, Yasmin A. Begum, Ashraful I. Khan, Abu S. G. Faruque, Nirod Chandra Saha, et al., "Impact of Rapid Urbanization on the Rates of Infection by *Vibrio cholerae* O1 and Enterotoxigenic *Escherichia coli* in Dhaka, Bangladesh," *PLOS Neglected Tropical Diseases* 5, no. 4 (2011): e999.

97. Mohammad H. Forouzanfar, Christopher J. L. Muray, Ashkan Afshin, Lily Alexander, Sten Biryukov, Michael Brauer, et al., "Global, Regional, and National Comparative Risk Assessment of 79 Behavioral, Environmental and Occupational, and

Metabolic Risks or Clusters of Risks in 195 Countries, 1990–2015: A Systematic Analysis for the Global Burden of Disease Study 2015," *Lancet* 388 (2016): 1659–1724; Pinar Keskin, Gauri Kartini Shastry, and Helen Willis, "Water Quality Awareness and Breastfeeding: Evidence of Health Behavior Change in Bangladesh," *Review of Economics and Statistics* 99, no. 2 (May 2017): 265–280; Syed Masud Ahmed, Timothy G. Evans, Hilary Standing, and Simeen Mahmud, "Harnessing Pluralism for Better Health in Bangladesh," *Lancet* 382 (2013): 1746–1755; Alayne M. Adams, Tanvir Ahmed, Shams El Arifeen, Timothy G. Evans, Tanvir Huda, and Laura Reichenbach, "Innovation for Universal Health Coverage in Bangladesh: A Call to Action," *Lancet* 382 (2013): 2104–2111; Shams El Arifeen, Aliki Christou, Laura Reichenbach, Ferdous Arfina Osman, Kishwar Azad, Khaled Shamsul Islam, et al., "Community-Based Approaches and Partnerships: Innovations in Health-Service Delivery in Bangladesh," *Lancet* 382 (2013): 2012–2026.

98. Institute for Health Metrics and Evaluation, "Global Burden of Disease Results Tool," 2013, http://ghdx.healthdata.org/gbd-results-tool.

99. Chowdhury et al., "Bangladesh Paradox," 1737; Hans Rosling, "The Bangladesh Miracle," Gapminder, Oct. 26, 2007, https://www.gapminder.org/videos/gapminder videos/gapcast-5-bangladesh-miracle/.

100. World Bank DataBank, "Urban Population," http://data.worldbank.org/indicator /SP.URB.TOTL?end=2015&start=1968.

101. Doug Bierend, "The Chaotic, Colorful Slums of the World's Most Overcrowded City," *Wired Magazine*, March 19, 2014, https://www.wired.com/2014/03/dhaka-slums -sebastian-keitel/.

102. Sonia R. Bhalotra, Alberto Diaz-Cayeros, Grant Miller, Alfonso Miranda, and Atheendar S. Venkataramani, "Urban Water Disinfection and Mortality Decline in Developing Countries," IZA Institute of Labor Economics Discussion Paper No. 10618 March 2017; Ayse Ercumen, Benjamin F. Arnold, Emily Kumpel, Zachary Burt, Isha Ray, Kara Nelson, and John M. Colford Jr., "Upgrading a Piped Water Supply from Intermittent to Continuous Delivery and Association with Waterborne Illness: A Matched Cohort Study in Urban India," *PLOS Medicine* 12, no. 10 (2015): e1001892.

103. Caroline van den Berg and Alexander Danilenko, *The IBNET Water Supply and Sanitation Performance Blue Book: The International Benchmarking Network for Water and Sanitation Utilities Databook* (Washington, DC: World Bank, 2011).

104. Esther Duflo, Michael Greenstone, Raymond Guiteras, and Thomas Clasen, "Toilets Can Work: Short and Medium Run Health Impacts of Addressing Complementarities and Externalities in Water and Sanitation," NBER Working Paper No. 21521, 2015; Marcella Alsan and Claudia Goldin, "Watersheds in Infant Mortality: The Role of Effective Water and Sewerage Infrastructure, 1880 to 1915," NBER Working Paper No. 21263, 2015.

105. Tove A. Larsen, Sabine Hoffmann, Christoph Lüthi, Bernhard Truffer, and Max Maurer, "Emerging Solutions to the Water Challenges of an Urbanizing World," *Science* 352, no. 6288 (2016): 928–933.

106. GBD Diarrheal Diseases Collaborators, "Estimates of Global, Regional, and National Morbidity, Mortality, and Aetiologies of Diarrhoeal Diseases: A Systematic Analysis for the Global Burden of Disease Study 2015," *Lancet Infectious Diseases* 17, no. 9 (2017): 909–948.

107. Thomas J. Bollyky, Christopher Troeger, Joseph Dieleman, and Robert Reneir, "The Role of Case-Management in Declining Diarrheal Disease Rates in Urban India" (forthcoming).

108. These countries are India, Nigeria, Democratic Republic of the Congo, Pakistan, Ethiopia, Kenya, Uganda, Niger, Bangladesh, and Tanzania. C. C. Unger, S. S. Salam, M. S. Sarker, R. Black, A. Cravioto, and S. El Arifeen, "Treating Diarrhoeal Disease in Children Under Five: The Global Picture," *Archives of Disease in Childhood* 99 (2014): 273–278; UNICEF, Global Databases, "Diarrhoea Treatment: Children Under 5 with Diarrhea Receiving Oral Rehydration Salts (ORS Packets or Pre-packaged ORS Fluids)—Percentage" (last update Dec. 2016), http://data.unicef.org.

109. David A. Leon, "Cities, Urbanization and Health," *International Journal of Epidemiology* 37 (2008): 4–8.

110. Demographia, *World Urban Areas*, 18.

111. Bairoch, *Cities and Economic Development*, 223–226.

112. Edward L. Glaeser, "A World of Cities: The Causes and Consequences of Urbanization in Poorer Countries," *Journal of the European Economic Association* 12, no. 5 (Oct. 2014): 1154–1199.

113. Edward Glaeser and J. Vernon Henderson, "Urban Economics for the Developing World: An Introduction," *Journal of Urban Economics* 98 (2017): 1–5.

114. Glaeser, "World of Cities," 1161.

115. Juan Pablo Chauvin, Edward Glaeser, Yueran Ma, and Kristina Tobio, "What Is Different about Urbanization in Rich and Poor Countries? Cities in Brazil, China, India and the United States," *Journal of Urban Economics* 98 (March 2017): 17–49.

116. Somik Vinay Lall, J. Vernon Henderson, and Anthony J. Venables, *African Cities: Opening Doors to the World* (Washington, DC: The World Bank, 2017), 74.

117. Glaeser, "World of Cities," 1155.

118. Demographia, *Demographia World Urban Areas*, 12th annual ed. (Belleville, IL: Demographia, 2016). 18.

119. Demographia, *Demographia World Urban Areas*, 19.

120. Paul Dorosh and James Thurlow, "Agriculture and Small Towns in Africa," *Agricultural Economics* 44, no. 4–5 (July–Sept. 2013): 449–459.

121. Robert D. Kaplan, "The Coming Anarchy: How Scarcity, Crime, Overpopulation, Tribalism, and Disease Are Rapidly Destroying the Social Fabric of Our Planet," *Atlantic Monthly*, Feb. 1994, 44–76.

122. Erik German, "Dhaka: Fastest Growing Megacity in the World," *PRI: Global Post*, Sept. 8, 2010.

123. Glaeser, *Triumph of the City*.

124. Wolfgang Fengler, "Can Rapid Population Growth Be Good for Economic Development?" World Bank (blog), April 15, 2010, http://blogs.worldbank.org/africa can/can-rapid-population-growth-be-good-for-economic-development; World Bank, *World Development Report 2009: Reshaping Economic Geography* (Washington, DC: The World Bank Group, 2009), 55–58.

125. Alex Ezeh, Oyinlola Oyebode, David Satterthwaite, Yen-Fu Chen, Robert Ndugwa, Jo Sartori, et al., "The History, Geography, and Sociology of Slums and the Health Problems of People Who Live in Slums," *Lancet* 389, no. 10068 (2017): 547–558.

126. Ezeh et al., "History, Geography, and Sociology," 553.

127. Glaeser, "World of Cities," 1187.

128. Ezeh et al., "History, Geography, and Sociology," 553.

129. Williamson, *Coping with City Growth*, 39, 53.

130. Szreter, *Health and Wealth*, 220–229; Williamson, *Coping with City Growth*, 272–274, 294–295, 298.

131. The data depicted in this figure are from Remi Jebwab, Luc Christiaensen, and Marina Gindelsky, "Demography, Urbanization, and Development: Rural Push, Urban Pull and…Urban Push?" *Journal of Urban Economics* 98 (2017). The African average shown in the figure includes data from ten countries: Central African Republic, Ethiopia, Kenya, Madagascar, Malawi, Burkina Faso, Ghana, Ivory Coast, Mali, and Senegal. The South and Southeast Asia average includes nine countries: Bangladesh, India, Pakistan, Sri Lanka, Indonesia, Malaysia, Myanmar, Philippines, and Thailand. The regional averages depicted are not population weighted.

132. Remi Jedwab and Dietrich Vollrath, "The Urban Mortality Transition and Poor Country Urbanization" (working paper, April 15, 2017), https://growthecon.com /assets/Jedwab_Vollrath_Web.pdf.

133. Christopher Dye, "Health and Urban Living," *Science* 319 (2008): 766–768.

134. John Bongaarts and John Casterline, "Fertility Transition: Is Sub-Saharan Africa Different?" *Population Development Review* 38, suppl. 1 (2013): 153–168.

135. E. M. Zulu, D. Beguy, A. C. Ezeh, P. Bocquier, N. J. Madise, J. Cleland, and J. Falkingham, "Overview of Migration, Poverty and Health Dynamics in Nairobi City's Slum Settlements," *Journal of Urban Health* 88, suppl. 2 (2011): S185–S99.

136. Jacques Emina, Donatien Beguy, Eliya M. Zulu, Alex C. Ezeh, Kanyiva Muindi, Patricia Elung'ata, et al., "Monitoring of Health and Demographic Outcomes in Poor Urban Settlements: Evidence from the Nairobi Urban Health and Demographic Surveillance System," *Journal of Urban Health* 88, suppl. 2 (2011): 200–218.

137. Montgomery et al., *Cities Transformed*, 209–212, 233.

138. Remi Jedwab and Dietrich Vollrath, "Urbanization without Growth in Historical Perspective," *Explorations in Economic History* 58 (2015): 1–21.

139. Paul Collier and Anthony J. Venables, "Urbanization in Developing Economies: The Assessment," *Oxford Review of Economic Policy* 33, no. 3 (2017): 355–372.

140. World Bank DataBank, "Improved sanitation facilities, urban (% of urban population)," http://data.worldbank.org/; UNICEF and World Health Organization, *Progress on Sanitation and Drinking Water—2015 Update and MDG Assessment* (Geneva: WHO, 2015), 56.

141. UNICEF and WHO, *Progress on Sanitation and Drinking Water*, 17.

142. Jedwab and Vollrath, "Urban Mortality Transition." See also Bert F. Hoselitz, "Generative and Parasitic Cities," *Economic Development and Cultural Change* 3, no. 3 (1955): 278–294; Bert F. Hoselitz, "Urbanization and Economic Growth in Asia," *Economic Development and Cultural Change* 6, no. 1 (1957): 42–54; Michael P. Todaro, "A Model of Labor Migration and Urban Unemployment in Less Developed Countries," *American Economic Review* 59, no. 1 (1969): 138–148.

143. Qimiao Fan and Martin Rama, "Seize the Opportunity to Make Dhaka a Great, Vibrant City," World Bank blog, July 19, 2017, http://blogs.worldbank.org/endpoverty insouthasia/seize-opportunity-make-dhaka-great-vibrant-city.

144. Mike Davis, *Planet of Slums* (New York: Verso, 2006), 23.

145. Jedwab and Vollrath, "Urban Mortality Transition," 13–15.

146. Ezeh et al., "History, Geography, and Sociology," 549.

147. UN-Habitat, "World Habitat Day 2014: Background Paper," http://unhabitat .org/wp-content/uploads/2014/07/WHD-2014-Background-Paper.pdf.

148. UN-Habitat, "State of the World Cities 2012/2013" (Nairobi, Kenya: UN-Habitat, 2013), 4 http://mirror.unhabitat.org/pmss/listItemDetails.aspx?publicationID=3387 &AspxAutoDetectCookieSupport=1.

149. Ezeh et al., "History, Geography, and Sociology," 549.

150. Joan Robinson, *Economic Philosophy* (New York: Penguin, 1962), 46.

151. Douglas Gollin, Remi Jedwab, and Dietrich Vollrath, "Urbanization with and without Industrialization," *Journal of Economic Growth* 21, no. 35 (2016): 35–70.

152. Rachel Heath and A. Mushfiq Mobarak, "Manufacturing Growth and the Lives of Bangladeshi Women," *Journal of Development Economics* 115 (2015): 1–15.

153. World Bank, "Bangladesh Development Update: Towards More, Better and Inclusive Jobs" World Bank Group Working Paper (Washington, DC: World Bank Group, 2017), 21–23; Kiran Stacey, "Bangladesh Garment-Making Success Prompts Fears for Wider Economy," *Financial Times*, Jan. 6, 2017.

154. Asian Development Bank and Bangladesh Bureau of Statistics, "The Informal Sector and Informal Employment in Bangladesh" (Mandaluyong City, Philippines: Asian Development Bank, 2012), https://www.adb.org/sites/default/files/publication /30084/informal-sector-informal-employment-bangladesh.pdf; Thomas Farole and Yoonyoung Cho, "Jobs Diagnostic: Bangladesh," World Bank Group Working Paper (Washington, DC: World Bank Group, 2017), vi.

155. Somik Vinay Lall, J. Vernon Henderson, and Anthony J. Venables, "Africa's Cities: Opening Doors to the World," World Bank Group Working Paper (Washington, DC: World Bank Group, 2017), 10; Somik V. Lall, "Renewing Expectations about Africa's Cities," *Oxford Review of Economic Policy* 33, no. 3 (2017): 521–539; Shohei Nakamura, Rawaa Harati Somik V. Lall, Yuri M. Dikhanov, Nada Hamadeh, William Vigil Oliver, et al., "Is Living in African Cities Expensive?" Policy Research Working Paper 7641 (Washington, DC: World Bank Group, 2016).

156. Joe Studwell, *How Asia Works: Success and Failure in the World's Most Dynamic Region* (London: Profile Books, 2014); Glaeser, "World of Cities," 1170; Council on Foreign Relations, "Poor World Cities: A Conversation with Edward Glaeser," Oct. 21, 2016, http://www.cfr.org/development/poor-world-cities-conversation-edward-glaeser /p38468.

157. Council on Foreign Relations, "Poor World Cities."

158. Bairoch, *Cities and Economic Development*, 466–467; Demographia, *Demographia World Urban Areas* (2016).

159. Ross Chainey, "Which Is the World's Most Polluted City?" *World Economic Forum*, June 25, 2015, https://www.weforum.org/agenda/2015/06/which-is-the-worlds-most -polluted-city/.

160. Abheet Singh Sethi, "Delhi's Pollution One-and-Half Times Worse Than Beijing," *Hindustan Times*, Dec. 29, 2015, http://www.hindustantimes.com/cities/delhi-s -pollution-one-and-half-times-worse-than-beijing/story-zGXWaA0sMG3nwTEeU59SaP .html.

161. Institute for Health Metrics and Evaluation, "Global Burden of Disease Results Tool," 2015, http://ghdx.healthdata.org/gbd-results-tool.

162. Susan Hanson, Robert Nicholls, N. Ranger, S. Hallegatte, J. Corfee-Morlot, C. Herweijer, and J. Chateau, "A Global Ranking of Port Cities with High Exposure to Climate Extremes," *Climate Change* 104, no. 1 (2011); 89–111.

163. Stephen Radelet, *The Great Surge: The Ascent of the Developing World* (New York: Simon and Schuster, 2015), 272; Gardiner Harris, "Borrowed Time on Disappearing Land: Facing Rising Seas, Bangladesh Confronts the Consequences of Climate Change," *New York Times*, March 29, 2014, https://www.nytimes.com/2014/03/29/world/asia/facing-rising-seas-bangladesh-confronts-the-consequences-of-climate-change.html.

164. Poppy McPherson, "Dhaka: The City Where Climate Refugees Are Already a Reality," *Guardian*, Dec. 1, 2015, https://www.theguardian.com/cities/2015/dec/01/dhaka-city-climate-refugees-reality.

165. Jeremy L. Wallace, *Cities and Stability: Urbanization, Redistribution, and Regime Survival in China* (Oxford: Oxford University Press, 2014), 56.

166. Edward L. Glaeser, Matt Resseger, and Kristina Tobio, "Inequality in Cities," *Journal of Regional Science* 49, no. 4 (2009): 617–646; Edward L. Glaeser and Bryce Millett Steinberg, "Transforming Cities: Does Urbanization Promote Democratic Change?" NBER Working Paper No. 22860, Nov. 2016, 6.

167. Wallace, *Cities and Stability*, 11.

168. National Intelligence Council, "Global Trends: Paradox of Progress" (Washington, DC: National Intelligence Council, Jan. 2017), 166, https://www.dni.gov/files/images/globalTrends/documents/GT-Main-Report.pdf.

169. Andrew R.C. Marshall and Manuel Mogato, "Philippine Death Squads Very Much in Business as Duterte Set for Presidency," *Reuters*, May 26, 2016, http://www.reuters.com/article/us-philippines-duterte-killings-insight-idUSKCN0YG0EB.

170. Nancy Birdsall, "Middle-Class Heroes," *Foreign Affairs*, March–April 2016.

171. Julfikar Ali Manik, Geeta Anand, and Russell Goldman, "Bangladeshi Troops Move to End Hostage Standoff," *New York Times*, July 1, 2016, https://www.nytimes.com/2016/07/02/world/asia/attackers-seize-hostages-and-detonate-explosives-in-bangladesh-restaurant.html.

172. "Mass Dissatisfaction: A Huge Protest in the Capital Against an Islamist Party and Its Leaders," *Economist*, Feb. 16, 2013, http://www.economist.com/news/asia/21571941-huge-protest-capital-against-islamist-party-and-its-leaders-mass-dissatisfaction; Eleanor Albert, "The Struggle Over Bangladesh's Future," interview of Alyssa Ayres, Council on Foreign Relations, July 25, 2016, http://www.cfr.org/bangladesh/struggle-over-bangladeshs-future/p38155.

173. International Monetary Fund, "Statement at the Conclusion of the IMF Mission for the Fifth and Sixth Reviews under the Extended Credit Facility (ECF) Arrangement

with Bangladesh," Press Release No. 15/103, March 10, 2015; "Businesses See Political Unrest Hitting Bangladesh's Image," *bdnews24.com*, March 3, 2015, http://bdnews24 .com/business/2015/03/02/businesses-see-political-unrest-hitting-bangladeshs -image. See also Shashank Bengali and Mohiuddin Kader, "Bangladesh's Long Political Crisis: Deaths and a Stilted Economy," *Los Angeles Times*, March 10, 2015, http: //www.latimes.com/world/asia/la-fg-bangladesh-political-crisis-20150310-story.html.

174. Eleanor Albert, "The Struggle Over Bangladesh's Future"; Sumit Ganguly and Ali Riaz, "Bangladesh's Homegrown Problem: Dhaka and the Terrorist Threat," *Foreign Affairs*, July 6, 2016, https://www.foreignaffairs.com/articles/bangladesh/2016 -07-06/bangladeshs-homegrown-problem.

175. William B. Milam, "The Real Source of Terror in Bangladesh," *New York Times*, May 19, 2016, https://www.nytimes.com/2016/05/20/opinion/the-real-source-of -terror-in-bangladesh.html.

176. Chowdhury et al., "Bangladesh Paradox."

177. Joseph Dieleman, Tara Templin, Nafis Sadat, Patrick Reidy, Abigail Chapin, Kyle Foreman, et al., "National Spending on Health by Source for 184 Countries between 2013 and 2040," *Lancet* 387, no. 10037 (June 18, 2016): 2521–2535.

178. Ramesh Govindaraj, Dhushyanth Raju, Federica Secci, Sadia Chowdhury, and Jean-Jacques Frere, *Health and Nutrition in Urban Bangladesh: Social Determinants and Health Sector Governance: Directions in Development* (Washington, DC: World Bank, 2018); Alayne M. Adams, Rubana Islam, and Tanvir Ahmed, "Who Serves the Urban Poor? A Geospatial and Descriptive Analysis of Health Services in Slum Settlements in Dhaka, Bangladesh," *Health Policy and Planning* 30 (2015): i32–i45; Nicola Banks, Manoj Roy, and David Hulme, "Neglecting the Urban Poor in Bangladesh: Research, Policy and Action in the Context of Climate Change," *Environment & Urbanization* 23, no. 2 (2011): 487–502.

179. Alyssa Ayres, "Political Polarization and Religious Extremism in Bangladesh," prepared statement before the Committee on Foreign Affairs, Subcommittee on Asia and the Pacific, United States House of Representatives 1st Session, 114th Congress, Council on Foreign Relations, http://i.cfr.org/content/publications/attachments /Ayres%20HFAC%20written%20statement%2004302015.pdf.

180. World Bank, *Migration and Remittances Factbook 2016* (Washington, DC: World Bank Group, 2016), 3.

Chapter 5: Diseases of Place

1. John Briscoe, "Hydropower for Me But Not for Thee: Why Poor Nations Deserve the Large Dams from Which the West Has Benefited," *The Breakthrough Institute*, https: //thebreakthrough.org/index.php/programs/energy-and-climate/hydropower-for-me

-but-not-for-thee; cited in Adam Bernstein, "John Briscoe, a Water-Resource Expert Who Championed Dams, Dies at 66," *Washington Post*, Nov. 17, 2014, www.washingtonpost .com/local/obituaries/john-briscoe-a-water-resource-expert-who-championed-dams -dies-at-66/2014/11/17/9742079c-6e74-11e4-ad12-3734c461eab6_story.html.

2. Brian Greenwood, "Manson Lecture: Meningococcal Meningitis in Africa," *Transactions of the Royal Society of Tropical Medicine and Hygiene* 93, no. 4 (1999): 341–353.

3. Felicity Thompson, "End of a Century Long Scourge?" *Bulletin of the World Health Organization* 89 (2011): 550–551.

4. Anaïs Colombini, Fernand Bationo, Sylvie Zongo, Fatoumata Ouattara, Ousmane Badolo, Philippe Jaillard, et al., "Costs for Households and Community Perception of Meningitis Epidemics in Burkina Faso," *Clinical Infectious Diseases* 49, no. 10 (2009): 1520–1525.

5. Patricia Akweongo, Maxwell A. Dalaba, Mary H. Hayden, Timothy Awine, Gertrude N. Nyaaba, Dominic Anaseba, et al., "The Economic Burden of Meningitis to Households in Kassena-Nankana District of Northern Ghana," *PLOS ONE* 8, no. 11 (2013): e79880, doi:10.1371/journal.pone.0079880.

6. Mary Moran, Nick Chapman, Lisette Abela-Oversteegen, Vipul Chowdhary, Anna Doubell, Christine Whittall, et al., *Neglected Disease Research and Development: The Ebola Effect*, G-FINDER Project (Sydney: Policy Cures, 2015), 14.

7. F. Marc LaForce and Jean-Marie Okwo-Bele, "Eliminating Epidemic Group A Meningococcal Meningitis in Africa through a New Vaccine," *Health Affairs* 30, no. 6 (2011): 1049–1057; Patrick Lydon, Simona Zipursky, Carole Tevi-Benissan, Mamoudou Harouna Djingarey, Placide Gbedonou, Brahim Oumar Youssouf, and Michel Zaffran, "Economic Benefits of Keeping Vaccines at Ambient Temperature during Mass Vaccination: The Case of Meningitis A Vaccine in Chad," *Bulletin of the World Health Organization* 92 (2013): 86–92.

8. Doumagoum M. Daugla, J. P. Gami, Kadidja Gamougam, Nathan Naibei, Lodoum Mbainadji, Maxime Narbé, et al., "Effect of a Serogroup A Meningococcal Conjugate Vaccine (PsA–TT) on Serogroup A Meningococcal Meningitis and Carriage in Chad: A Community Study," *Lancet* 383, no. 9911 (2014): 40–47; Kathy Neuzil, "Breaking the Paradigm: How an Essential Vaccine Was Fast-Tracked," PATH (blog), Jan. 8, 2015, https://blog.path.org/2015/01/menafrivac-infant-prequal/.

9. Donald McNeill, "New Meningitis Strain in Africa Brings Calls for More Vaccines," *New York Times*, July 31, 2015, https://www.nytimes.com/2015/08/01/health /new-meningitis-strain-in-africa-brings-call-for-more-vaccines.html.

10. "Serum Institute to Launch 4 Vaccines, Enter US, Europe Market," *Times of India*, Dec. 7, 2017; Amanda Glassman and Miriam Temin, "Eliminating Meningitis across Africa's Meningitis Belt," in *Millions Saved: New Cases of Proven Success in Global Health* (Washington, DC: Center for Global Development, 2016).

11. The Carter Center, "Guinea Worm Case Totals," https://www.cartercenter.org/health/guinea_worm/case-totals.html.

12. Institute for Health Metrics and Evaluation, "Global Burden of Disease 2015," http://ghdx.healthdata.org/gbd-results-tool.

13. Michel Boussinesq, "A New Powerful Drug to Combat River Blindness," *Lancet*, Jan. 17, 2018, http://www.thelancet.com/journals/lancet/article/PIIS0140-6736(18)30101-6/fulltext.

14. Bill and Melinda Gates Foundation, "Enteric and Diarrheal Diseases: Strategy Overview,"   http://www.gatesfoundation.org/What-We-Do/Global-Health/Enteric-and-Diarrheal-Diseases.

15. "Final Trial Results Confirm Ebola Vaccine Provides High Protection against Disease," *World Health Organization*, Dec. 23, 2016, http://www.who.int/mediacentre/news/releases/2016/ebola-vaccine-results/en/.

16. Nuno Rodrigues Faria, Raimunda do Socorro da Silva Azevedo, Moritz U. G. Kraemer, Renato Souza, Mariana Sequetin Cunha, Sarah C. Hill, et al., "Zika Virus in the Americas: Early Epidemiological and Genetic Findings," *Science* (March 24, 2016).

17. World Bank DataBank, "GDP per Capita (Current US$)," http://data.worldbank.org/indicator/NY.GDP.PCAP.CD?locations=NE.

18. United Nations Development Programme, "Human Development Data (1990–2015)," http://hdr.undp.org/en/data.

19. Joseph L. Dieleman, Tara Templin, Nafis Sadat, Patrick Reidy, Abigail Chapin, Kyle Foreman, et al., "National Spending on Health by Source for 184 Countries between 2013 and 2040," *Lancet* 387 (2016): 2521–2535.

20. United Nations Development Programme, "Human Development Data (1990–2015)," http://hdr.undp.org/en/data.

21. IHME Country Profiles, "Niger," http://www.healthdata.org/niger.

22. Institute for Health Metrics and Evaluation, "Global Burden of Disease 2015."

23. World Bank DataBank, "Fertility Rate, Total (Births per Woman)," http://data.worldbank.org/indicator/SP.DYN.TFRT.IN?locations=NE.

24. John F. May, Jean-Pierre Guengant, and Thomas R. Brooke, "Demographic Challenges of the Sahel," *Population Reference Bureau*, 2015, http://www.prb.org/Publications/Articles/2015/sahel-demographics.aspx.

25. Thomas L. Friedman, "Out of Africa," *New York Times*, April 13, 2016, A25.

26. Somini Sengupta, "Heat, Hunger and War Force Africans Onto a 'Road on Fire,'" *New York Times*, Dec. 15, 2016, https://www.nytimes.com/interactive/2016/12/15/world/africa/agadez-climate-change.html.

27. Marc Levinson, *The Box: How the Shipping Container Made the World Smaller and the World Economy Bigger*, 2nd ed. (Princeton, NJ: Princeton University Press, 2016).

28. Peter Tinti and Tuesday Reitano, *Migrant, Refugee, Smuggler, Saviour* (London: Hurst, 2016), 92.

29. Ben Taub, "We Have No Choice," *New Yorker*, April 10, 2017, 36.

30. International Organization for Migration, *Niger Flow Monitoring Points (FMP) Statistical Report—Overview* (2016), http://www.globaldtm.info/dtm-niger-flow-monitoring-statistical-report-november-2016/.

31. International Organization for Migration, *Niger Flow Monitoring Points (FMP)*.

32. "IOM Records Over 60,000 Migrants Passing through Agadez, Niger between February and April 2016," IOM Niger, May 27, 2016, https://www.iom.int/news/iom-records-over-60000-migrants-passing-through-agadez-niger-between-february-and-april-2016.

33. International Organization for Migration, "Missing Migrants Project," https://missingmigrants.iom.int.

34. Taub, "We Have No Choice."

35. Tinti and Reitano, *Migrant, Refugee, Smuggler, Saviour*, 167.

36. Adam Nossiter, "Crackdown in Niger Fails to Deter Migrant Smugglers," *New York Times*, Aug. 20, 2015, https://www.nytimes.com/2015/08/21/world/africa/migrant-smuggling-business-is-booming-in-niger-despite-crackdown.html.

37. Tim Cocks and Edward McAllister, "Africa's Population Boom Fuels 'Unstoppable' Migration to Europe," *Reuters*, Oct. 13, 2016, http://www.reuters.com/article/us-europe-migrants-africa-analysis-idUSKCN12D1PN.

38. Tinti and Reitano, *Migrant, Refugee, Smuggler, Saviour*, 92, 149.

39. Maggie Fick, James Politi, and Duncan Robinson, "Migration: Reversing Africa's Exodus," *Financial Times*, Nov. 6, 2016; Cocks and McAllister, "Africa's Population Boom."

40. Michelle Hoffman, "Seeking Alternatives for Niger's People Smugglers," *UNHCR News*, Aug. 9, 2017, http://www.unhcr.org/news/latest/2017/8/59882a2a4/seeking-alternatives-nigers-people-smugglers.html.

41. Taub, "We Have No Choice," 36; Lisa Schlein, "Dramatic Drop in Number of Migrants Crossing the Sahel to Europe," *VOA News*, Oct. 12, 2017.

42. Fick, Politi, and Robinson, "Migration."

43. Kevin O'Neill, *Family and Farm in Pre-Famine Ireland: The Parish of Killashandra* (Madison: University of Wisconsin Press, 2003), 166, 187.

44. Massimo Livi-Bacci, *A Concise History of World Population*, 5th ed. (Chichester: Wiley-Blackwell, 2012), 63.

45. Robert E. Kennedy, *The Irish, Emigration, Marriage, and Fertility* (Berkeley: University of California Press, 1973), 32–35.

46. Kennedy, *Irish, Emigration, Marriage*, 46–48; Cormac Ó Gráda and Philem B. Boyle, "Fertility Trends, Excess Mortality, and the Great Irish Famine," *Demography* 23, no. 4 (1986): 543–562.

47. Ó Gráda and Boyle, "Fertility Trends," 547–548, 560.

48. Kennedy, *Irish, Emigration, Marriage*, 46–49.

49. Timothy J. Hatton and Jeffrey G. Williamson, *What Fundamentals Drive Future Migration* (Canberra: Center for Economic Policy Research, Australian National University, 2002).

50. Kennedy, *Irish, Emigration, Marriage*, 27.

51. Kennedy, *Irish, Emigration, Marriage*, 214.

52. Jean-Claude Chesnais, *The Demographic Transition: Stages, Patterns, and Economic Implications* (Oxford: Oxford University Press, 1992); Timothy J. Hatton and Jeffrey G. Williamson, "Demographic and Economic Pressure on Emigration out of Africa," *Scandinavian Journal of Economics* 105, no. 3 (2003): 465–486, 466.

53. Timothy J. Hatton and Jeffrey G. Williamson, "What Drove the Mass Migrations from Europe in the Late Nineteenth Century?" *Population and Development Review* 20, no. 3 (Sep. 1994): 533–559, 544–545, 550.

54. Richard A. Easterlin, "Influences in European Overseas Emigration before World War I," *Economic Development and Cultural Change* 9, no. 3 (1961): 331–351.

55. Hatton and Williamson, "What Drove the Mass Migrations," 537, 542–543.

56. Gordon H. Hanson and Craig McIntosh, "Is the Mediterranean the New Rio Grande? US and EU Immigration Pressures in the Long Run," *Journal of Economic Perspectives* 30, no. 4 (2016): 1–25.

57. Michael Clemens, forthcoming untitled paper (Washington, DC: Center for Global Development).

58. Robert I. Woods, Patricia A. Watterson, and John H. Woodward, "The Causes of Rapid Infant Mortality Decline in England and Wales, 1861–1921, Part I," *Population Studies* 42, no. 3 (1988): 343–366.

59. Hatton and Williamson, "What Drove the Mass Migrations."

60. Hatton and Williamson, "Demographic and Economic Pressure."

61. Hein de Haas, "Turning the Tide? Why Development Will Not Stop Migration," *Development and Change* 38, no. 5 (2007): 819–841.

62. Sebastian Mallaby, "Globalization Resets," *Finance and Development* 53, no. 4 (2016): 6–10.

63. David S. Reher, "Economic and Social Implications of the Demographic Transition," *Population and Development Review* 37, suppl. s1 (2011): 11–33.

64. Henrik Urdal, "The Devil in the Demographics: The Effect of Youth Bulges on Domestic Armed Conflict, 1950–2000," World Bank Social Development, Working Paper No. 14, 2004; Michael A. Clemens and David McKenzie, "Why Don't Remittances Appear to Affect Growth?" World Bank Policy Research, Working Paper No. 6856, 2014.

65. World Bank, *Migration and Development: A Role for the World Bank Group* (Washington, DC: World Bank Group, 2016).

66. Internal Displacement Monitoring Centre, Norwegian Refugee Council, *Global Estimates 2015: People Displaced by Disasters* (Geneva: Norwegian Refugee Council, 2015), 5, 17.

67. World Bank, *Migration and Development*, 13.

68. Reher, "Economic and Social Implications," 24.

69. Reginald Appleyard, "International Migration Policies: 1950–2000," *International Migration* 39, no. 6 (2001): 9.

70. Appleyard, "International Migration Policies"; Béla Lipták, *A Testament to a Revolution* (College Station: Texas A&M University College Press, 2007); Michael A. Clemens and Justin Sandefur, "A Self-Interested Approach to Migration Crises: Push Factors, Pull Factors, and Investing in Refugees," *Foreign Affairs*, Sept. 27, 2015, https://www.foreignaffairs.com/articles/central-europe/2015-09-27/self-interested -approach-migration-crises; Marjoleine Zieck, "The 1956 Hungarian Refugee Emergency, an Early and Instructive Case of Resettlement," *Amsterdam Law Forum* 5, no. 2 (2013): 45–63.

71. United Nations, *International Migration Policies: Government Views and Priorities* (New York: United Nations, 2013), 44, table 2.1.

72. Appleyard, "International Migration Policies."

73. Josh Dawsey, "Trump Derides Protections for Immigrants from 'Shithole' Countries," *Washington Post*, Jan. 12, 2018.

74. Renee Stepler, "World's Centenarian Population Projected to Grow Eightfold by 2050," Pew Research Center, April 21, 2016, http://www.pewresearch.org/fact-tank /2016/04/21/worlds-centenarian-population-projected-to-grow-eightfold-by-2050/.

75. Peter H. Diamandis and Steven Kotler, *Abundance: The Future Is Better Than You Think* (New York: Simon & Schuster), 198–199.

76. Council on Foreign Relations, "Cell Phones without Factories: A Conversation with Tyler Cowen," Dec. 7, 2016, https://www.cfr.org/event/cell-phones-without-factories -conversation-tyler-cowen-international-economic-development.

Chapter 6: The Exoneration of William H. Stewart

1. Douglas Martin, "William H. Stewart Is Dead at 86; Put First Warnings on Cigarette Packs," *New York Times*, April 29, 2008, A17.

2. Centers for Disease Control and Prevention, "Trends in Current Cigarette Smoking among High School Students and Adults, United States, 1965–2014," http:// www.cdc.gov/tobacco/data_statistics/tables/trends/cig_smoking/index.htm.

3. Michael Stobbe, *Surgeon General's Warning: How Politics Crippled the Nation's Doctor* (Berkeley: University of California Press, 2014), 128–139; Martin, "William H. Stewart Is Dead at 86"; Matt Schudel, "William H. Stewart; Surgeon General Condemned Smoking," *Washington Post*, April 27, 2008, http://www.washingtonpost .com/wp-dyn/content/article/2008/04/26/AR2008042602246.html.

4. Martin, "William H. Stewart Is Dead at 86"; Nellie Bristol, "William H. Stewart," *Lancet* 372 (2008): 110.

5. Michael Specter, "One of Science's Most Famous Quotes Is False," *New Yorker*, Jan. 5, 2015, http://www.newyorker.com/tech/elements/william-stewart-science-erroneous -quote.

6. The initial citation to Stewart's purported remarks at NIAID referenced a 1969 Stewart speech, but that particular speech actually occurred in 1968. Brad Spellberg and Bonnie Taylor-Blake, "On the Exoneration of Dr. William H. Stewart: Debunking an Urban Legend," *Infectious Diseases of Poverty* 2, no. 3 (2013): 3.

7. Specter, "One of Science's Most Famous Quotes."

8. Gerald B. Pier, "On the Greatly Exaggerated Reports of the Death of Infectious Diseases," *Clinical Infectious Diseases* 47, no. 8 (2008): 1113–1114; Frank MacFarlane Burnet, "Viruses," *Scientific American* 184, no. 5 (1951): 51.

9. William H. Stewart, "A Mandate for State Action," in *Proceedings of the 65th Annual Meeting of the Association of State and Territorial Health Officers* (Washington, DC: Association of State and Territorial Health Officers, 1967).

10. Centers for Disease Control and Prevention, "Antibiotic/Antimicrobial Resistance," https://www.cdc.gov/drugresistance/.

11. William H. Stewart, "Areas of Challenge for the Future," in *Schools of Public Health: Changing Institutions in a Changing World: Three Papers Presented on the Occasion of the*

Dedication of the Ernest Lyman Stebbins Building (Baltimore: Johns Hopkins University School of Hygiene and Public Health, 1968).

12. Fitzhugh Mullan, *Plagues and Politics: The Story of the U.S. Public Health Service* (New York: Basic Books, 1989), 153.

13. Partners in Health, "Press Conference Held on Treating Non-Communicable Disease in Poor Populations," http://www.pih.org/press/press-conference-held-on -treating-non-communicable-disease-in-poor-populati.

14. Edward Glaeser and Wentao Ziong, "Urban Productivity in the Developing World," NBER Working Paper No. 23279 (2017); Raj Chetty, M. Stepner, S. Abraham, S. Lin, B. Scuderi, N. Turner, et al., "The Association between Income and Life Expectancy in the United States, 2001–2014: Association between Income and Life Expectancy in the United States," *JAMA* 315, no. 16 (2016): 1750–1766.

15. Laura B. Nolan, David E. Bloom, and Ramnath Subbaraman, "Legal Status and Deprivation in India's Urban Slums: An Analysis of Two Decades of National Sample Survey Data," IZA Discussion Papers, No. 10639 (2017); Somik Vinay Lall, J. Vernon Henderson, and Anthony J. Venables, "Africa's Cities: Opening Doors to the World," World Bank Group Working Paper (Washington, DC: World Bank Group, 2017), 121–132, 152; Sebastian Galiani and Ernesto Schargrodsky, "Property Rights for the Poor: Effects of Land Titling," *Journal of Public Economics* 94, nos. 9–10 (2010): 700– 729; Brookings Institution, *Foresight Africa: Top Priorities for the Continent in 2017* (Washington, DC: Brookings Press, 2017), 65.

16. World Bank, *Providing Water to Poor People in African Cities Effectively: Lessons from Utility Reforms* (Washington, DC: World Bank, 2016), xiii–xv, 18, 20–21, 30.

17. Glaeser and Ziong, "Urban Productivity," 42.

18. Lant Pritchett, *The Rebirth of Education: Schooling Ain't Learning* (Washington, DC: Center for Global Development, 2103), 13–21; Justin Sandefur, "Measuring the Quality of Girls' Education across the Developing World," Center for Global Development (blog), Oct. 12, 2016, https://www.cgdev.org/blog/measuring-quality-girls-education -across-developing-world; UNECSO, *Global Education Monitoring Report 2016, Education for People and Planet: Creating Sustainable Futures for Us All* (Paris: UNESCO, 2016), 195.

19. International Monetary Fund, Regional Economic Outlook, *Sub-Saharan Africa: Navigating Headwinds* (Washington DC: IMF, 2015), 25.

20. UNICEF Eastern and Southern Africa Regional Office, *Improving Quality Education and Children's Learning Outcomes and Effective Practices in the Eastern and Southern Africa Region: Report for UNICEF ESARO* (UNICEF, 2016), xi, https://www.unicef.org /esaro/ACER_Full_Report_Single_page_view.pdf.

21. Mauricio Romero, Justin Sandefur, and Wayne Aaron Sandholtz, "Can Outsourcing Improve Liberia's Schools?" (Center for Global Development Working Paper 462, 2017).

22. Some experts have suggested that the improvement may be less than this study suggests and may be the result of other factors, such as classroom size and better-trained teachers, rather than private management. Steven J. Klees, "Liberia's Experiment," National Center for the Study of Privatization in Education, Working Paper No. 235, Oct. 26, 2017, http://ncspe.tc.columbia.edu/center-news/working-paper -liberias-experiment/.

23. Caerus Capital, *The Business of Education in Africa* (2016), 12–17, https://edafri careport.caeruscapital.co/.

24. Deon Filmer, Jeffrey S. Hammer, Lant H. Pritchett, "Weak Links in the Chain: A Diagnosis of Health Policy in Poor Countries," *World Bank Research Observer* 15 (2000): 199–224.

25. "Why Developing Countries Must Improve Primary Care," *Economist*, Aug. 24, 2017.

26. James Macinko and Matthew J. Harris, "Brazil's Family Health Strategy—Delivering Community-Based Primary Care in a Universal Health System," *New England Journal of Medicine* 372 (2015): 2177–2181.

27. AMPATH Kenya, "Our Model," http://www.ampathkenya.org/our-model; Thomas J. Bollyky, *New, Cheap, and Improved: Assessing the Promise of Reverse and Frugal Innovation to Address Noncommunicable Diseases* (New York: Council on Foreign Relations, 2015).

28. Julio Frenk, "Bridging the Divide: Global Lessons from Evidence-Based Health Policy in Mexico," *Lancet* 368 (2006): 954–961.

29. Richard Cash, "Step by Step: The Path to Ending Child Mortality," Harvard T. H. Chan School of Public Health, filmed Oct. 9, 2013, https://www.youtube.com /watch?v=EkUfhVfrXHY.

30. Vital Strategies, "Vital Strategies launches Resolve, a New $225 Million Global Health Initiative," press release, Sept. 12, 2017, http://www.vitalstrategies.org/vital -stories/vital-strategies-launches-resolvenew-225-million-global-healthinitiative/.

31. Angus S. Deaton and Robert Tortora, "People in Sub-Saharan Africa Rate Their Health and Health Care among the Lowest in the World," *Health Affairs* 34, no. 3 (2015): 519–527; Shannon L. Lövgren, Trisa B. Taro, and Heather L. Wipfli, "Perceptions of Foreign Health Aid in East Africa: An Exploratory Baseline Study," *International Health* 6, no. 4 (2014): 331–336.

32. UNECSO, *Global Education Monitoring Report 2016*, 193–203, 281.

33. Thomas J. Bollyky and David Fidler, "Has a Global Tobacco Treaty Made a Difference?" *Atlantic*, Feb. 28, 2015, https://www.theatlantic.com/health/archive/2015 /02/has-a-global-tobacco-treaty-made-a-difference/386399/.

34. Sonia Angell, Jessica Levings, Andrea Neiman, Samira Asma, and Robert Merritt, "How Policy Makers Can Advance Cardiovascular Health," in *Promoting Cardiovascular Health Worldwide*, ed. Valentin Fuster, Jagat Narula, Rajesh Vedanthan, and Bridget B. Kelly (New York: Scientific American Custom Media, 2014), 24–29.

35. Kai-Alexander Kaiser, Caryn Bredenkamp, and Roberto Magno Iglesias, *Sin Tax Reform in the Philippines: Transforming Public Finance, Health, and Governance for More Inclusive Development* (Washington, DC: World Bank, 2016).

36. Kathryn Grace, Frank Davenport, Chris Funk, and Amy M. Lerner, "Child Malnutrition and Climate in Sub-Saharan Africa: An Analysis of Recent Trends in Kenya," *Applied Geography* 35, nos. 1–2 (2012): 405–413.

37. World Bank, "Which Coastal Cities Are at Highest Risk of Damaging Floods? New Study Crunches the Numbers," Aug. 19, 2013, http://www.worldbank.org/en /news/feature/2013/08/19/coastal-cities-at-highest-risk-floods.

38. Richard Haass, *A World in Disarray: American Foreign Policy and the Crisis of the Old Order* (New York: Penguin Press, 2017), 226–255.

39. Christopher Hamlin, "Cholera Forcing: The Myth of the Good Epidemic and the Coming of Good Water," *American Journal of Public Health* 99 (2009): 1946–1954.

Index

An "f" following the page number indicates a figure.